OBSTETRICS AND GYNECOLOGY ADVANCES

THE THIN PINK LINE

REGULATING REPRODUCTION

OBSTETRICS AND GYNECOLOGY ADVANCES

Additional books and e-books in this series can be found on Nova's website under the Series tab.

OBSTETRICS AND GYNECOLOGY ADVANCES

THE THIN PINK LINE

REGULATING REPRODUCTION

CAROL LYNN CURCHOE BURTON, PHD

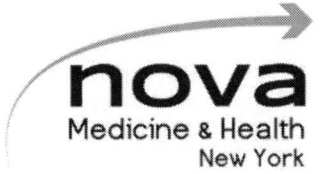

Copyright © 2021 by Nova Science Publishers, Inc.

All rights reserved. No part of this book may be reproduced, stored in a retrieval system or transmitted in any form or by any means: electronic, electrostatic, magnetic, tape, mechanical photocopying, recording or otherwise without the written permission of the Publisher.

We have partnered with Copyright Clearance Center to make it easy for you to obtain permissions to reuse content from this publication. Simply navigate to this publication's page on Nova's website and locate the "Get Permission" button below the title description. This button is linked directly to the title's permission page on copyright.com. Alternatively, you can visit copyright.com and search by title, ISBN, or ISSN.

For further questions about using the service on copyright.com, please contact:
Copyright Clearance Center
Phone: +1-(978) 750-8400   Fax: +1-(978) 750-4470   E-mail: info@copyright.com.

NOTICE TO THE READER

The Publisher has taken reasonable care in the preparation of this book, but makes no expressed or implied warranty of any kind and assumes no responsibility for any errors or omissions. No liability is assumed for incidental or consequential damages in connection with or arising out of information contained in this book. The Publisher shall not be liable for any special, consequential, or exemplary damages resulting, in whole or in part, from the readers' use of, or reliance upon, this material. Any parts of this book based on government reports are so indicated and copyright is claimed for those parts to the extent applicable to compilations of such works.

Independent verification should be sought for any data, advice or recommendations contained in this book. In addition, no responsibility is assumed by the Publisher for any injury and/or damage to persons or property arising from any methods, products, instructions, ideas or otherwise contained in this publication.

This publication is designed to provide accurate and authoritative information with regard to the subject matter covered herein. It is sold with the clear understanding that the Publisher is not engaged in rendering legal or any other professional services. If legal or any other expert assistance is required, the services of a competent person should be sought. FROM A DECLARATION OF PARTICIPANTS JOINTLY ADOPTED BY A COMMITTEE OF THE AMERICAN BAR ASSOCIATION AND A COMMITTEE OF PUBLISHERS.

Additional color graphics may be available in the e-book version of this book.

Library of Congress Cataloging-in-Publication Data

ISBN: 978-1-53619-150-9

Published by Nova Science Publishers, Inc. † New York

*To our daughter, Soleil Elyse Burton.
Our stars are other people's suns that we can see at night,
and our sun is just a star in someone else's night sky.
May you grow up in a world where your choices and reproductive
freedoms are not curtailed by the laws of men.*

CONTENTS

First Foreword   xi
    Allison K. Rodgers

Second Foreword   xv
    Natalie M. Crawford

Preface   xix
    Carol Lynn Curchoe Burton

Acknowledgments   xxi

Chapter 1	Medical Bondage	1
	The History of the Speculum and Fistula Surgery	*1*
	"Educational" Pelvic Exams	*8*
	HeLa Cells: The Immortal Legacy of Henrietta Lacks	*12*
	Skeletons in the Closet: Human Zoos and Imperial Collections	*15*
Chapter 2	Birth Control	21
	Eugenics and Ethical Lapses in the Quest for Hormonal Birth Control	*21*
	Griswold vs. Connecticut (1965)	*23*
	The Colorado Experiment	*24*

	Medication Abortions and Access on the Internet	28
	Period Poverty	30
Chapter 3	Coitus	33
	Contagious Diseases Act	33
	Premarital Blood Tests	34
	Marriage Annulment and Impotence	36
Chapter 4	Sterilization	39
	Eugenic Sterilization	41
	Chemical and Surgical Castration	43
	Access to Endometrium Ablation and Tubal Ligations	45
Chapter 5	Parturition	47
	The Royal Roots of "Back Labor"	47
	Episiotomy and Interventions	48
	The Husband Stitch	53
	Shackled and Separated: Parturition in Prison	53
	Midwives	55
	Pregnancy Crisis Centers	57
	Racial Disparities in the USA	59
Chapter 6	Gender	65
	The Origin of Female and Male Reproductive Tracts	65
	Development of the Reproductive Tracts	67
	Genetics, Sex, and Gender	70
	Official Documents	74
	Intersex Timeline	76
	Conversion Therapy	76
	Sex Selection	78

Chapter 7	Genital Alteration	**81**
	Genital Cutting	*81*
	Sex Reassignment Surgery	*83*
	Barriers to Sex Reassignment Surgery	*90*
	Denial of Gender-Affirming Care to Armed Services Veterans	*91*
Chapter 8	Assisted Reproductive Technology	**93**
	Assisted Reproductive Technologies (ART)	*93*
	Reproductive Tissue Donation	*96*
	Artificial Insemination	*100*
	Illegal Embryos	*107*
	Personhood Bills	*117*
Chapter 9	Research and Development	**119**
	Human Reproductive Experimentation	*119*
	Chimeras—How Much Human DNA Is Too Much?	*122*
	14 Days: The Limit of Human Life in the Lab	*124*
	Procuring Fetal Tissue for Research	*125*
References		**129**
About the Author		**135**
Index		**137**

First Foreword

Allison K. Rodgers, MD

I have always been a champion of educating women about their bodies and helping them understand and take control of their health. As a board-certified Obstetrician/Gynecologist and Reproductive Endocrinologist, I am in a unique position to have been trained in all areas of women's health, along with the ultra-specialized field of infertility. Using my voice as a TikTok and Instagram creator, as well as the medical contributor on the Beat Infertility Podcast has shown me how much people crave to know, understand, and advocate for themselves! The author, Dr. Carol Lynn (Curchoe) Burton, and I crossed paths on this shared mission of educating and empowering women. She has come to this mission from a different path, as a reproductive biologist with a basic-science background and PhD, training to end up at the same endpoint; to help women, help themselves.

While modern-day healthcare is based on science, facts, and evidence-based approaches, there are dark hidden pasts, that many do not know about, that have helped us get to this point of modern medicine, science, and technology. If you are reading this, you have benefited from some of these egregious practices that did advance our understanding of science but have harmed many people along the way.

In the infamous musical Hamilton, we are introduced to an American Hero, and realize when we take a deeper look, he was flawed and made mistakes. Just like Alexander Hamilton, our reproductive history is not as honorable and straight forward as we all were taught. *The Thin Pink Line: Regulating Reproduction*, is a truly eye-opening reminder of our past. Many of these unfathomable events seem so unethical and out-of-line based on today's values.

In this intriguing collection of reproductive topics ranging from the birth of modern gynecology, to future reproductive directions, Dr. Carol Lynn (Curchoe) Burton seeks to not only educate us about our mistakes of the past but pushes us to think about the ethics of our future. Will we look back and wonder, "what were we thinking?" There is a delicate balance, as a society, between allowing patient autonomy to make decisions about what is best for themselves and making decisions for them to protect them from "harm."

The Thin Pink Line: Regulating Reproduction, has reminded me of some deplorable areas of our reproductive history that I have personally witnessed. I have been the delivering obstetrician to an incarcerated woman, shackled to a bed during labor. An armed guard was the only non-medical person present to make sure that she did not escape during labor. I have cared for a patient who delivered alone on the floor of her prison cell, four months early, to a baby who did not survive, because the warden did not believe she was in pain. I have done basic science research on endometriosis and chlamydia, working with HeLa cells, which were stolen from a young African American mother during her fight with cervical cancer. I have worked with instruments designed and named after famous gynecologists who developed surgical advances on unanesthetized teenage slaves. I have had to surgically remove and then replace female genital mutilation for a patient who did not want to have normal genital anatomy for fear that she would never be an acceptable wife. I have cared for a patient who was such a shame to her husband and family after getting pregnant with a third daughter that she decided to terminate the pregnancy and presented to me for gender selection to avoid shame to her family for not producing a son. When I write that you personally have benefited, it is

First Foreword

because all of us have; vaccines, pharmaceuticals, surgical techniques, technological advances that originated from unethical origins are the norm, not the exception.

Coming from a place of rapid technological advances in the laboratory and procedures such as *in vitro* fertilization, Dr. Carol Lynn (Curchoe) Burton poses questions for us to consider about the current and future reproductive ethical decisions. Does reproductive health need more or less regulation? Who should be deciding?

Dr. Carol Lynn (Curchoe) Burton's *The Thin Pink Line: Regulating Reproduction* is a brave and honest look at where we have been, so we can figure out where we want to go. You will be thinking about these topics long after you have finished the last page. Everyone in science, as well as everyone who has a vagina and those who love someone with a vagina should read this book.

Allison K. Rodgers, MD
Board certified obstetrician and Gynecologist & Reproductive
Endocrinology and Infertility
Medical contributor for Beat Infertility Podcast
Women's Health Advocate

SECOND FOREWORD

Natalie M. Crawford, MD, MSCR, FACOG

Women's health has been regulated and politicized for much longer than we like to admit. When we look back through our own history, the truth is both alarming and eye opening. The use of women's health and reproduction as a political tool has simplified the issue down to abortion access and care. And despite the importance of this topic, and the relevance to modern life, the history of women's care is so much more than one single political issue. Many of us don't know the roots of racism and misogyny in medicine and reproductive care. Many of us don't want to acknowledge the past.

As a fertility physician, I see first-hand how the history of women's health plays a role in our everyday life. This is because reproduction is not talked about. From menstrual cycles, to infertility and miscarriage. The culture of silence and ignorance, which was a part of society long before women started leading conversations, is so ingrained in human behavior that an active movement is needed to discuss the past and change the future. As technology advances faster than research, we must understand the ethical principles that guide us as a field.

Honestly, there are parts of this book that are hard for me to read as a gynecologist. Things I know are true, and things I know that I wish were in the past, but sadly are not completely. I have seen women die from lack of medical care, I have taken care of patients who have been victims of female genital mutilation, I have seen the discrimination and hate laid at the feet of a trans person, I've watched how we treat our incarcerated, and I've had patients sterilized by the government who had no idea the procedure was done. I am a woman who believes in education and empowerment. But this is not just our history, it is also our present.

Dr. Curchoe Burton, a reproductive physiologist and senior clinical embryologist, has watched the first stages of life unfold in a dish in the lab. She has seen the ethical debate that exists in the reproductive world when it comes to research, legality of embryos, personhood, and the advancement of technology. If you ever sit in a lab and watch the first cells of human life divide, then you know – there is art in this science. But the responsibility to protect this beauty becomes your burden. We must not let ignorance be the guiding light regulating female reproduction by politicians and those with other motives. In *The Thin Pink Line*, Dr. Curchoe Burton has given life to something more – a telling of the past, present, and future with precision and an absolute attention to detail, as I know reflects her role overseeing life in the embryology lab.

> "Depending on who you ask, assisted reproduction is either one of the most or least regulated industries in the US."
> Carol Lynn Curchoe, PhD

The reproductive world is undergoing an evolution. There is high interest from tech companies and money being funneled into an industry of patient care. The largest network of fertility clinics in the US is led not by physicians, scientists, or embryologists, but by businessmen, and the people who are behind the industry advancing the science in our own IVF labs are all coming from outside medicine. At face value, advancement is always good. More money will be put into development and acquisition and new technology. But respecting research and upholding ethical principles is essential for our own society's growth. In order to do this, we must collectively understand the history of how we came to be as a field, the origins of women's health, and how reproduction has been, and continues to be, regulated.

Dr. Natalie M. Crawford, MD, MSCR, FACOG

PREFACE

Carol Lynn Curchoe Burton

When you picked up this book, you may have been expecting to read about the history of *Roe v. Wade* as the 50th anniversary of this historic decision is reached or about how abortion case law impacts patient care. Perhaps you are expecting to read about the hundreds of state laws that have been passed[1] to strangle access to safe, legal abortion care and the numerous clinics that have been shuttered due to these laws. The landmark 1973 Supreme Court *Roe v. Wade* ruling established that our constitutional right to privacy "is broad enough to encompass a woman's decision whether or not to terminate her pregnancy." This right was reaffirmed in 1991 in *Planned Parenthood v. Casey*.

I, like many of you, am incredibly anxious that the untimely passing of Justice Ruth Bader Ginsberg, rushed confirmation of Justice Amy Coney Barrett, and the conservative Supreme Court majority that directly threatens *Roe v. Wade* and *Planned Parenthood v. Casey,* yet I specifically avoided writing about federal legality of abortion care. Why?

Many constitutional law scholars believe a doctrine called "stare decisis" that promotes consistent, reliable, and predictable development of

---

[1] An Overview of Abortion Laws, Guttmacher Institute. https://www.guttmacher.org/state-policy/explore/overview-abortion-laws

the law, while assuring the public of the court's integrity, will prevent *Roe v. Wade* and *Planned Parenthood v. Casey* from being overturned. Precedent plays an important role in stability in our democracy. Disagreeing with the prior decision—and the court has emphasized this on several occasions—is not enough to overturn the precedent.

While I *am* certain that I could fill a book's worth of words about access to abortion, I'm not entirely positive that my anxiety and worry would not bias my research and writing, and I am equally uncertain that there are any new insights to garner from my apprehension that have not been spoken before by Elizabeth Cady Stanton, Margaret Sanger, Gloria Steinem, and dozens of other notable advocates both historical and contemporary in the fight for women's rights.

Many fine works have been written about abortion access[2], and this substantial topic tends to overshadow all of the other insidious and sometimes invisible ways that reproduction is regulated. By avoiding what is arguably the largest topic in reproduction, I can bring you a critical examination of the pervasive tension existing between good, ethical patient care and the regulation of various aspects of reproduction, from birth control to sterilization, to episiotomies and the "husband stitch," to "educational" pelvic exams, shackling laboring convicts, gender-affirming surgery, human embryo research, assisted reproduction, and much more.

The Thin Pink Line: Regulating Reproduction is intended to educate a wide audience of womynx, men, femmes, gender non-conforming folks, uterus owners, and everyone in between. It has a specific intersectional focus on the impact that the current reproductive regulatory framework has on disenfranchised groups, such as people of color, LQBTQ individuals, and the lower socioeconomic strata. By dissecting a myriad of issues of consent and access, my goal is to provide a historical perspective and help spur on generations to come.

---

[2] *Roe v. Wade*: Selected full-text books and articles. https://www.questia.com/library/controversial-topics/roe-v-wade.

ACKNOWLEDGMENTS

Why should you or I, or anyone write a book? There is a sacred place in the world for authors. Our words echo down the generations, and can have impact in other places and at other times, than the here and now. Writing is a lonely process, but the end result, is an opportunity, a chance encounter, the promise that a young person somewhere, at some point far in the future, and through any time or space, has a chance to make friends with my mind. Writing bends the space time continuum. Perhaps the greatest accomplishment in the history of humankind is the written word. Connecting generations in thought.

I have always loved books. When I was very young, I would write pages and pages of description- no plot, no story, no characters just description of environments. As I developed into a scientist, I learned the central tenant of research "publish or perish." If it's not published and peer-reviewed, it's like it never even happened. I learned to organize my work with the goal of publishing early on, and as one of the few folks who loves to research and write, this became a valued skill among my peers and colleagues.

But I was never happy "just" writing scientific papers. Soon, I turned my creative mind to spinning thrilling, fictional yarns with a science-y plot twist. I won the Wasatch Iron Pen (Utah Arts Festival, 2013) award for *In Bloom*, a short story about family values, veterinary medicine, and fetal reduction. I collected my short, creepy stories into a book, and pitched and pitched it, suffering 100 or so rejections, before self-publishing *The Tip Jar* (ISBN-10: 1304896668).

I outlined another book idea, exploring the etymology of common words, but stopped writing it after the first few chapters, maybe I'll pick that one back up someday.

When I got the idea for the *Thin Pink Line: Regulating Reproduction*, I knew - this was the book I, and I alone, was meant to write. A reflection of everything I've read, studied, and lived my whole life. This book would not have been possible without the countless people who helped mentor me along my journey to becoming a scientist and encouraged me to write. I can't thank enough the folks who have supported me along this long journey; my family- CJ and Soleil Burton, my parents and siblings. My best friends Rachel, Sara, Peijean, Caroline, Judy, Elisabeth, Jody, Stacy, and THEIR parents, who have always been our biggest cheerleaders. My lifelong mentors and friends; Sheenah Mische, Josh Baxt, Ann George, Cindy Loomis, Mary Migliorelli, Ann Mackin, and Charles Bormann. The friends and editors that helped to polish this final work and provided critical comments; Julie Swearingen, Lindsy Floyd, and Dona Mapston. Thank you for the amazing cover art Jenya Armen!! Thanks to my publisher Nova Science Books for accepting the pitch for this important work. Thank you to the fabulous, fierce physicians who wrote the forewords; doctors Allison Rodgers and Natalie Crawford. Lastly, to my junior trainees and mentees; for always believing in me, trusting me, and allowing me to mentor you.

Chapter 1

MEDICAL BONDAGE

THE HISTORY OF THE SPECULUM AND FISTULA SURGERY

On Tuesday, April 17th, 2018, a statue of J. Marion Sims was removed from the distinguished place of honor where it stood since 1934, in New York's Central Park, directly across from the New York Academy of Medicine. The story of Sims is a complicated one, as his legacy and celebrated discoveries in medicine, are tainted by practices that we now view as abhorrent.

J. Marion Sims[3] is known as the "Father of Gynecology" for his role in developing treatments and devices for gynecology, such as the modern speculum and fistula surgery. His *Clinical Notes on Uterine Surgery*, written in 1866 and the only clinical book he ever wrote, was a masterpiece and served to separate gynecology from obstetrics as a specialty. His book is remarkable for its accurate description of the fertile period in relation to the menstrual cycle, 50 years before it was rediscovered and really understood. Sims's records also detailed a successful case of artificial insemination.

---

[3] *The Story of My Life*, J. Marion Sims, 1884. https://archive.org/stream/storyofmylif00sims #page/n3/mode/2up.

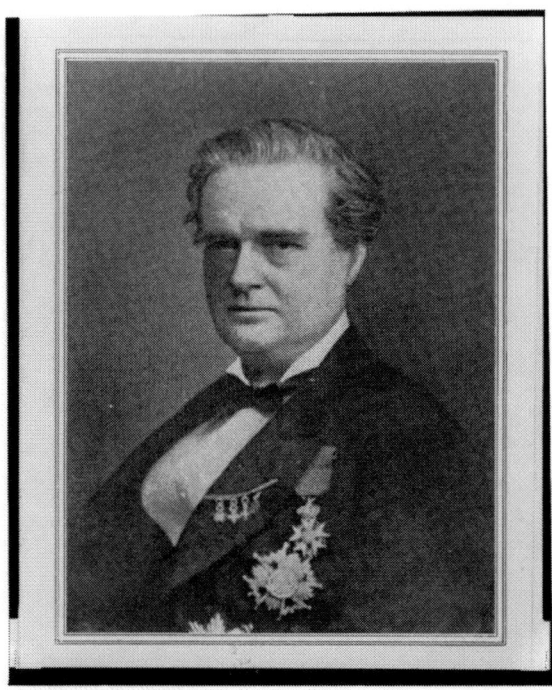

Image source: Wikimedia Commons.
https://commons.wikimedia.org/wiki/File:J._Marion_Sims,_head-and-shoulders_portrait,_facing_slightly_left_LCCN98504112.jpg.

Figure 1. J. Marion Sims, The Father of Gynecology: A complex historical figure whose actions (although they undoubtedly benefit us all), are considered to be abhorrent by today's standards.

Later, in 1868, he addressed the New York County Medical Society on the subject.

"The Microscope as an Aid in the Diagnosis and Treatment of Sterility." He advocated the importance of demonstrating spermatozoa in the semen. He complained that he "was misrepresented, maligned and positively abused both here and abroad" for his insistence on semen studies, and cited *The Medical Times and Gazette,* which charged that "this dabbling in the vagina with speculum and syringe was incompatible with decency and self-respect."[4]

While Sims was ahead of his time in many ways, many of his practices are viewed today as ethically abhorrent. For example, he developed the surgery for fistula—an unnatural opening between the bladder and vagina or rectum and vagina—by performing multiple experimental surgeries on un-anesthetized, enslaved Black teenage girls.

In his autobiography Sims wrote, "I got three or four more to experiment on, and there was never a time that I could not, at any day, have had a subject for operation. But my operations all failed ... this went on, not for one year, but for two and three, and even four years." Unlike the careful record keeping of the horrific Nazi medical experiments during the Holocaust, Sims's victims went unnamed, except for three: Anarcha, Betsey, and Lucy, all of whom were teenagers.

Anesthesia itself was just coming into use[5] during the time that Sims was perfecting his surgical technique to repair fistulas—the wounds between the bladder and vaginal or vagina and rectum—caused by protracted labor. Ether as an anesthetic was available as early as the beginning of 1842.

The population most vulnerable to fistula are malnourished girls. Rarely seen now in western societies, fistula is still common in cultures where children are forced into marriage and where malnutrition and underdevelopment of the bone structure of the pelvis compounds the risks of teenage (or younger) pregnancy.[6]

The removal of Sims's statue in 2018 came 24 years after SisterSong[7] coined the term "reproductive justice" as meaning "the human right to maintain personal bodily autonomy, have children, not have children, and parent the children we have in safe and sustainable communities" in 1994.

---

[4] "The History of Human Fertility, Donald Robert Johnston, MD, CM. https://www.fertstert.org/article/S0015-0282%2816%2934860-9/pdf.
[5] "first successful public demonstration of ether anaesthesia for a surgical operation, performed on October 16, 1846 in Boston/Massachusetts." https://www.ncbi.nlm.nih.gov/pubmed/9090947.
[6] http://www.halftheskymovement.org/
[7] "Reproductive Justice," SisterSong. https://www.sistersong.net/reproductive-justice/

The modern legal precedent for "simple" consent[8] was written in 1914, establishing a patient's "right to determine what shall be done with his body," just after Sims performed his surgical experimentation on enslaved and un-sedated persons from 1845-1849.

Although informed consent for clinical treatment has become a pillar of contemporary medical practice that has not always been the case, and to this day "informed consent" is an ever-evolving concept, complicated by practical consideration that rarely ever reaches the theoretical "ideal."[9] In the 1950s the notion evolved into an obligation for physicians to disclose details[10] about treatment in a process of informed consent, and in 1975 it evolved yet to obligate physicians disclose the information that a "reasonable person" would want to know in a similar situation.[11]

We view J. Marion Sims's actions today as running afoul of informed consent in medicine. Did he protect the patient from assault and battery in the form of unwanted medical interventions, prevent unwanted procedures, protect autonomous decision-making, and support patient defined goals?

It is likely that Anarcha, Lucy, and Betsey (or any of the other unnamed women) were not given the opportunity or disclosed sufficient details for them to make an informed choice. It is certain that they could not freely refuse the treatment plan, as Sims owned them, and they would have had no value to another owner, reeking of urine and feces, and being unable to reproduce further.

Today, women consenting to gynecological procedures *still* describe feeling forced to sign lengthy, convoluted consent forms,[12] perhaps under

---

[8] *Schloendorff v. Society of New York Hospital.* Vol. 211 N.Y. 125, 105 N.E. 921914.

[9] Hall, Daniel E et al. "Informed consent for clinical treatment." *CMAJ : Canadian Medical Association journal = journal de l'Association medicale canadienne* vol. 184,5 (2012): 533-40. doi:10.1503/cmaj.112120 https://www.ncbi.nlm.nih.gov/pmc/articles/PMC3307558/.

[10] Berg JW, Appelbaum P, Lidz C, et al. The legal requirements for disclosure and consent: History and current status. In: Informed consent: legal theory and clinical practice. 2nd ed New York (NY): Oxford University Press; 2001. p. 41–74.

[11] *Canterbury* v. *Spence.* Vol. 464 F.2d 772D.C. Cir. 1972.

[12] Why do women consent to surgery, even when they do not want to? An interactionist and Bourdieusian analysis. Dixon-Woods M, Williams SJ, Jackson CJ, Akkad A, Kenyon S, Habiba M. Soc Sci Med. 2006 Jun; 62(11):2742-53.
Women's accounts of consenting to surgery: is consent a quality problem? Habiba M, Jackson C, Akkad A, Kenyon S, Dixon-Woods M. Qual Saf Health Care. 2004 Dec; 13(6):422-7.

the duress of a time crunch or the threat of withholding needed treatment unless they are signed fully (and not modified). I discuss this in greater detail in Chapter 5: Parturition.

Versions of the gynecological speculum have been found in medical texts dating back to the Greek physician Galen in 130 A.D. and have shown up in archaeological digs as far back as 79 A.D. in Pompeii. However, in Sims's day, physicians would have examined women's genitals hesitantly, under their skirts, without actually seeing them, because it was considered to be improper and indecent. In Sims's autobiography he wrote, "If there was anything I hated, it was investigating the organs of the female pelvis." Sims would not have undergone any sort of specialized training before practicing medicine on humans. After graduating from South Carolina College at 21, he interned with the county's only physician, whose daughter he subsequently married, then completed a three-month course at Charleston Medical College, before going on to study at the Jefferson Medical College in Philadelphia for just one more year (1834-5). He was then a qualified doctor.

Sims operated on these children without anesthesia partly due to a lack of his own training, as patients occasionally died of overdoses. However, the cost of providing anesthesia would have also been a consideration, as well as the commonly held notion that Black women could bear the pain. The surgeries were so gruesome in their horror and pain that other physicians and assistants lost their desire to assist Sims during the surgeries, perhaps in holding the patients down during the surgeries or hearing their cries as they endured repeated operations.

Coincidentally, during the time Sims was perfecting his technique, Dr. Samuel Cartwright published a paper in 1851 entitled, "Report On The Diseases and Physical Peculiarities Of The Negro race" in *The New Orleans Medical and Surgical Journal*, a reputable scholarly publication.[13]

The paper's main conjecture was the existence of drapetomania, a disease that would cause slaves to attempt to flee captivity. If a slave

---

[13] Cartwright, Samuel A. 1851. Report on the diseases and physical peculiarities of the Negro race. http://heinonline.org/HOL/Page?handle=hein.slavery/disphypcnr0001&id=1&collection=slavery

appeared "sulky and dissatisfied without cause," it was a warning sign of imminent flight. His prescription to stop the disease from fully taking over the slave was, as he writes in his own words, "whipping the devil out of them" as a "preventative measure." As a remedy for this "disease," the doctor made running physically impossible by prescribing the removal of both big toes. I shudder at the use of the word "prescribing" in this context.

He also coined a mental illness called dysaesthesia aethiopica, which supposedly made slaves lazy in their work. He further conjectured that for treatment of dysaesthesia aethiopica; "The best means to stimulate the skin is, first, to have the patient well washed with warm water and soap; then, to anoint it all over in oil, and to slap the oil in with a broad leather strap; then to put the patient to some hard kind of work in the sunshine." The horrors of the treatment slaves had to endure under the thin guise of medical language cannot be overstated.

To this day, inaccurate and racially biased pain management means that whites are more likely to be prescribed strong pain[14] medications for equivalent ailments to Blacks. Women are also routinely undertreated for pain. A 2001 study published in the *Journal of Law, Medicine & Ethics*[15] found that doctors frequently incorrectly believe that women have a "natural capacity to endure pain" and possess more coping mechanisms for pain, presumably due to what we have to endure in childbirth.

So many women have reported intolerably painful hysteroscopies (a procedure where a catheter is passed through the cervix, and the uterus is inflated to inspect it, and possibly take a biopsy or remove other abnormal tissue), and felt that doctors have not been truthful about the prospect of pain and not counseled appropriately to make an informed decision on the

---

[14] Kelly M. Hoffman, Sophie Trawalter, Jordan R. Axt, M. Norman Oliver. "Racial bias in pain assessment." Proceedings of the National Academy of Sciences Apr 2016, 201516047; DOI: 10.1073/pnas.1516047113 https://www.pnas.org/content/early/2016/03/30/1516 047113.abstract.

[15] Hoffmann, Diane E. and Tarzian, Anita J., The Girl Who Cried Pain: A Bias Against Women in the Treatment of Pain (2001). Available at SSRN: https://ssrn.com/abstract=383803 or http://dx.doi.org/10.2139/ssrn.383803.

availability of pain control including anesthesia, that in the UK a group of survivors has formed the Campaign Against Painful Hysteroscopy.[16]

The group has pressured the authorities to pay more attention to pain management during the common gynecological procedure of hysteroscopy. The British Society for Gynaecological Endoscopy issued a statement in December 2018[17]: "It is important that women are offered, from the outset, the choice of having the procedure performed as a day case procedure under general or regional anesthetic. [...] It is important that the procedure is stopped if a woman finds the outpatient experience too painful for it to be continued."

I can relate to the women's stories through my own experience of having a Foley balloon catheter inserted into my cervix during my labor, it was then slowly inflated and pulled through my cervical canal over approximately 12 hours overnight. I was crawling up the bed in so much pain, trying to get away from my (male) physician, but at the same time trying to endure anything it took to get my daughter birthed safely. The next morning a (female) nurse burst in to take my vitals, which were all over the map because I was in so much pain, and immediately offered me morphine for pain management. I was not offered it or told it was even a possibility until then. Those 12 hours were agonizing, excruciating, and traumatizing. I was burdened with the memory of my medical torture for many months after, as I also learned how to be a first-time mother to a colicky, low-birthweight, premature infant.

Another example of the confluence of stereotypes (racial and gender) and commonly held medical myths, is that women in general, but perhaps more so Black women who present with symptoms of endometriosis are often misdiagnosed with pelvic inflammatory disease (PID), a condition that is sexually transmitted. Research on the illness in Black women and other women of color is not as substantial as documented research in white patients.

One of the ways that doctors can make an accurate diagnosis is through exploratory laparoscopic surgery. The decision to move forward

---

[16] Hysteroscopy Action website, https://www.hysteroscopyaction.org.uk/.
[17] https://www.bsge.org.uk/.

with this surgery lies solely with the doctor's validation of the patient's complaints of pain.

"Educational" Pelvic Exams

In 2015, 52 million pelvic examinations were performed in the United States alone. How do doctors learn to perform a pelvic exam? How can it be, that like in so much of healthcare, we are both routinely overtreating non-symptomatic individuals and under-educating and undertreating symptomatic women?

In 45 states, doctors and medical students are legally allowed to practice pelvic exams on patients who are under anesthesia without being granted explicit consent to do so. The practice is explicitly outlawed in Hawaii, Illinois, Virginia, Oregon, and California.[18] In California, unauthorized pelvic exams are a misdemeanor and grounds for loss of license. Pelvic exams without consent are still widely practiced in countries worldwide, including Canada.[19]

Shawn Barnes writes in the journal *Obstetrics & Gynecology* (2012):[20]

> "In obstetrics and gynecology, I encountered the first act of medical training that left me ashamed. For 3 weeks, four to five times a day, I was asked to, and did, perform pelvic examinations on anesthetized women, without specific consent, solely for the purpose of my education.
>
> Typically, this would unfold as follows: I would be assigned a gynecologic surgery case on which to scrub in. I would be required to go meet the patient beforehand and introduce myself as "the medical student on the team" or some such vague statement of my role in the procedure, without mentioning a pelvic examination. I then would follow the patient

---

[18] "Non-consensual Pelvic Examinations," John Kasprak, Senior Attorney. https://www.cga.ct.gov/2004/rpt/2004-R-0512.htm

[19] "Pelvic exams without consent still possible under new guidelines: report," *The Globe and Mail,* March 2012. https://www.theglobeandmail.com/life/health-and-fitness/pelvic-exams-without-consent-still-possible-under-new-guidelines-report/article534399/

[20] Barnes, Shawn S. "Practicing Pelvic Examinations by Medical Students on Women Under Anesthesia: Why Not Ask First?" *Obstetrics & Gynecology.* 1 October 2012.

into surgery. Once anesthesia was administered and the patient was asleep, the attending or resident would ask me to perform a pelvic examination on the patient for educational purposes. To my shame, I obeyed."

In some states, signing a "consent to treat" form in some teaching hospitals allows doctors to perform a medically unnecessary test, such as a pelvic exam. In several surveys of medical students, including one at the University of Oklahoma,[21] the majority of students said they had performed a pelvic exam on an unconscious woman.

Dr. Jennifer Goedken argues in "Pelvic Examinations Under Anesthesia: An Important Teaching Tool,"[22] that from a clinician's viewpoint the teaching of pelvic examinations is equal to any other examination skill, from lungs, to heart, to big toe. She argues that the sexual mores of society place restrictions on the ability of physicians to provide care, when really it's only the patients who view the genitals as being "sensational."

"To the obstetrician gynecologist, female genitalia do not, and arguably should not, be anything but routine in the same way that a plumber views a sink or drain pipes," said Dr. Jennifer Goedken.

Goedken rightly notes that it is impossible for patients to have knowledge of activities that take place when they are under anesthesia. This is particularly important because students often give pelvic exams when the patient is under anesthesia for non-gynecological treatments. Meaning this exam is given outside of the true scope of care for the patient, simply as a teaching opportunity.

In another example, Janine, a nurse in Arizona, checked into the hospital for stomach surgery in 2017. Before the procedure, she told her physician that she did not want medical students to be directly involved. But after the operation, Janine recalled that when the anesthesia wore off a resident came by to inform her that she had gotten her period—the resident

---

[21] Schniederjan S, Donovan GK. "Ethics versus education: pelvic exams on anesthetized women." J Okla State Med Assoc. 2005 Aug; 98(8):386-8. PMID: 16206868.

[22] Goedken J. "Pelvic examinations under anesthesia: an important teaching tool." J Health Care Law Policy. 2005;8(2):232-9. PMID: 16471020.

had noticed while conducting a pelvic exam. Janine had a history of sexual abuse and trying to figure out what happened while she was under anesthesia caused her to have panic attacks. Unfortunately, many similar stories have been shared on Twitter and aggregated under the hashtag #MeTooPelvic. The state of Utah passed legislation in 2019 banning pelvic examinations on patients under anesthesia who have not knowingly given consent to the procedure. SB188[23] closed a loophole where patients technically gave consent, but it was disguised among the many papers a patient signs before surgery. SB188 now requires consent to be given in a large font and in a separate form in order for a pelvic exam to be performed under anesthesia, and it applies to both men and women.

Certainly, pelvic exams need to be taught to doctors as well as any other skill. Reproductive-related anatomy and physiology have historically led to undertreatment of urinary incontinence and sexual dysfunction, and there is evidence that postpartum prolapse (rectocele, cystocele, urethrocele and enterocele—each a type of pelvic organ prolapse) is still undertreated[24] in the US, partially because women are not educated about these conditions or the signs and symptoms to look for. Sexual health education in the US is lacking at all levels,[25] starting with youth, through the childbearing and postmenopausal years.

In France, pelvic rehabilitation after childbirth is sponsored by the French government and preliminary data show significantly reduced incontinence and pelvic pain at nine months after giving birth.[26] Birth control and abortion are also both legal *and* subsidized by the government.

Recently, there has been a slew of bills banning unauthorized pelvic exams in 11 states. Maryland, Utah, New York, and Delaware passed laws

---

[23] https://le.utah.gov/~2019/bills/static/SB0188.html
[24] Clifford, Christen, "My vagina was badly injured after giving birth. Why was getting help do hard?", *The Guardian*, December 2017. https://www.theguardian.com/us-news/commentisfree/2017/dec/28/vaginal-health-post-partum-maternity-rectocele.
[25] Hall, Kelli Stidham et al. "The State of Sex Education in the United States." *The Journal of adolescent health : official publication of the Society for Adolescent Medicine* vol. 58,6 (2016): 595-7. doi:10.1016/j.jadohealth.2016.03.032. https://www.ncbi.nlm.nih.gov/pmc/articles/PMC5426905/.
[26] Lundberg, Claire, "The French Government Wants to Tone My Vagina," Slate, February 2012. https://slate.com/human-interest/2012/02/postnatal-care-in-france-vagina-exercises-and-video-games.html

mandating informed consent, joining six other states to mandate clear, specific, and universally employed standards for consent processes for breast, pelvic, urogenital, prostate, and rectal exams.

While some conditions in the US seem to be undertreated, in general the routine "bimanual pelvic examination" (examining the pelvis with two hands, usually with two fingers of one hand on the inside through the vaginal canal while the other hands presses the organs down from the abdomen) seems to in and of itself be in question as an appropriate screening tool. Frequent routine bimanual examinations may partly explain why US rates of (unnecessary) ovarian cystectomy and hysterectomy are more than twice as high as rates in European countries, where the use of the pelvic examination is limited to *symptomatic* women.

Justifications gynecologists typically offer for doing the pelvic exam—screening for a sexually transmitted infection and cervical cancer, early detection of ovarian cancer, and evaluating a woman for hormonal contraception—either do not require a bimanual exam or are not supported by research.[27,28] The American College of Obstetrics and Gynecology has stated that the decision to perform a pelvic examination should be a shared decision between the patient and her obstetrician–gynecologist or other gynecologic care provider and based on medical history and symptoms.[29]

Racial and socioeconomic disparities have been noted in pelvic exam training. In private insurance clinics, medical students mostly observe residents perform gynecological procedures, whereas, it has been noted that exams primarily for patients on Medicaid or the uninsured seem to encourage more "hands on" experience. In 2003, Dr. Ira Silver-Isenstadt coauthored a study titled "Don't Ask, Don't Tell," published in the

---

[27] Qaseem A, Humphrey LL, Harris R, Starkey M, Denberg TD. "Screening pelvic examination in adult women: a clinical practice guideline from the American College of Physicians." Clinical Guidelines Committee of the American College of Physicians. Ann Intern Med 2014;161:67–72.

[28] Guirguis-Blake JM, Henderson JT, Perdue LA. Periodic screening pelvic examination: evidence report and systematic review for the US Preventive Services Task Force. *JAMA* 2017;317:954–66.

[29] "The Utility of and Indications for Routine Pelvic Examination," The American College of Obstetricians and Gynecologists, October 2018. https://www.acog.org/Clinical-Guidance-and-Publications/Committee-Opinions/Committee-on-Gynecologic-Practice/The-Utility-of-and-Indications-for-Routine-Pelvic-Examination

American Journal of Obstetrics and Gynecology. He surveyed 401 students at five Pennsylvania medical schools and found that 90 percent had performed pelvic exams on anesthetized patients.[30] In one small survey,[31] 62 percent of patients said they *would* consent to medical students doing pelvic examinations. So why aren't they plainly asked?

The majority of patients want to help medical students learn but expect consent to be obtained. However, medical faculty members often argue that patients implicitly consent to being enlisted in medical teaching when visiting a teaching hospital, or that consent for one gynecological procedure encompassed consent for any additional, related exams. Even in France (seemingly a beacon of gender parity, sexual health, and consent), pelvic and rectal exams are given to patients under anesthesia without their explicit consent.[32] Legislative action may well be the only way to affect a step-change in the culture of this widely accepted practice by medical institutions worldwide.

HeLa Cells: The Immortal Legacy of Henrietta Lacks

In 1951, at the age of 31, the woman Henrietta Lacks ceased to exist, but the cells of her cervix live on to this day. A tissue biopsy obtained for diagnostic evaluation was sent to Dr. George O. Gey's tissue culture laboratory at Johns Hopkins (Baltimore, Maryland).

---

[30] "Don't ask, don't tell: A change in medical student attitudes after obstetrics/gynecology clerkships toward seeking consent for pelvic examinations on an anesthetized patient," *American Journal of Obstetrics & Gynecology,* Volume 188, Issue 2, p575-579, February 1, 2003. https://www.ajog.org/article/S0002-9378(02)71415-4/fulltext.

[31] Wainberg, Sara et al. "Teaching pelvic examinations under anaesthesia: what do women think?." *Journal of obstetrics and gynaecology Canada: JOGC = Journal d'obstetrique et gynecologie du Canada*: JOGC vol. 32,1 (2010): 49-53. doi:10.1016/S1701-2163(16)34404-8.

[32] "TRIBUNE: Never again vaginal examination on sleeping patients without prior consent," Dix Lunes, February 2015. http://10lunes.com/2015/02/tribune-plus-jamais-de-toucher-vaginal-sur-patientes-endormies-sans-consentement-prealable/#_edn1

These cells (dubbed HeLa for the first two letters of her first and last names) became the first ever "immortal" (meaning they could be endlessly propagated in a culture dish) human cell culture line.

Before Mrs. Lacks[33] tissue sample was successfully cultured, over 30 other patients' cervical cancer tissue samples had been tested. All of them failed to grow. Mrs. Lacks aggressive adenocarcinoma of the cervix was so virulent that it turned her internal organs into solid masses of tumors within months of her initial complaints.[34]

---

[33] Jones, H. W. "Record of the first physician to see Henrietta Lacks at the Johns Hopkins Hospital: history of the beginning of the HeLa cell line." *Am J Obstet Gynecol* 1997. 176:227S–228S.

[34] Lucey, B et al. "Henrietta Lacks, HeLa Cells, and Cell Culture Contamination" https://meridian.allenpress.com/aplm/article/133/9/1463/64025/Henrietta-Lacks-HeLa-Cells-and-Cell-Culture "Small, white, and firm nodules were observed throughout both the thoracic and abdominal cavities, including the surfaces of the peritoneum, the entire length of the intestines, and the surface of the liver. Furthermore, both the pleural surface and the superior surface of the diaphragm (right side more than the left side) were covered with nodules, as were the lung, liver parenchyma, and the pericardium. The nodules varied slightly in size, measuring from 8 mm in diameter on the peritoneal surface to 1 cm in the lung parenchyma. However, the largest mesenteric lymph node infiltrated with tumor was 6 cm in length. Small tumor nodules, 3 mm in diameter, were seen in each adrenal gland. At the apex of the right ventricle, a tumor nodule approximately 1 cm in diameter protruded into the lumen. Relatively little necrosis was seen in any of the nodules.

A large subcapsular hematoma was present at the superior pole of the right kidney and a tumor nodule had grown into the capsule. Bilaterally, the ureters, calyces, and pelves were markedly dilated, consistent with severe hydronephrosis. The left ureter was involved in a mass of tumor just inside the brim of the pelvis, while a tumor mass near the posterior wall of the bladder entangled the right ureter. The bladder itself was adherent to the anterior abdominal wall. Many small nodules were seen on the bladder mucosa, and the external surface was nearly a solid mass of tumor.

The right ureter was dilated within 4 cm of the bladder, where the dilatation ceased abruptly. At this level, the circumference of the ureter was 14 mm; distally, the right ureter had been left intact and a probe passed with some difficulty down to the bladder. The probe could not be passed through the left ureter to the bladder, although both ureteral openings appeared patent from within the bladder. Closer examination revealed that the left ureter was dilated to the bladder wall, at which point a mass of tumor on the external surface caused the obstruction. The bladder was partially surrounded by nodular masses of tumor that penetrated the bladder wall, particularly in the trigone area. The bladder was not especially dilated. Tumor was seen infiltrating the wall of the vagina and friable masses of tumor replaced the cervix. The uterus was approximately normal in size and covered with tumor nodules, while the fallopian tubes and ovaries were obliterated by clusters of tumor nodules. A mass of tumor surrounded the iliac veins, and the area of the right iliac vein appeared to have tumor entering its lumen. Focal uremic diphtheritic colitis was also noted."

Gey and colleagues published data[35] with HeLa cells in 1952, reporting the "evaluation *in vitro* of the growth potential of normal, early intra-epithelial, and invasive carcinoma from a series of cases of cervical carcinoma." Only the HeLa cells established themselves in "continuous roller-tube cultures for almost a year." It was not until 1975, when a random encounter with HeLa cells by the brother-in-law of a family friend that their provenance came to light.

Due to the unusual virulence of these cells, it is no wonder they have been continuously propagated for *seven decades*, allowing physicians and scientists to make astonishing discoveries. Research using HeLa cells has led to significant advances in medical science, such as the polio vaccine,[36] human telomerase (an enzyme that protects chromosomes from degrading), and significant advances in cancer mitigation among many, many others.

Johns Hopkins was the only hospital in the area to treat Black patients at the time. They issued a statement after the 2010 popular book by Rebecca Skloot, *The Immortal Life of Henrietta Lacks*, stating:

> "It's important to note that at the time the cells were taken from Mrs. Lacks's tissue, the practice of obtaining informed consent from cell and tissue donors was essentially unknown among academic medical centers."

Although the modern legal precedent for "simple" consent was written in 1914, it had not been widely implemented 40 years later.

We now have the Common Rule,[37] the Federal Policy for Protection of Human Subjects, which governs research on humans, tissues, and genetic material. The current US system of protection for human research subjects is heavily influenced by an older document, known as the Belmont Report, which was written in 1979 by the National Commission for the Protection

---

[35] Gey, G. O., W. D. Coffman, and M. T. Kubicek. "Tissue culture studies of the proliferative capacity of cervical carcinoma and normal epithelium." Cancer Res 1952. 12:264–265.
[36] Scherer, W. F., J. T. Syverton, and G. O. Gey. "Studies on the propagation *in vitro* of poliomyelitis viruses." J Exp Med 1953. 97:695–710.
[37] Federal Policy for the Protection of Human Subjects ('Common Rule'). https://www.hhs.gov/ohrp/regulations-and-policy/regulations/common-rule/index.html.

of Human Subjects of Biomedical and Behavioral Research. The Belmont Report outlines the basic ethical principles in research involving human subjects. The Common Rule offers additional protections for pregnant women, human fetuses, and neonates (subpart B); additional protections for prisoners (subpart C); and additional protections for children (subpart D). The original Common Rule was written decades before anyone imagined what we can now learn from DNA and public records analysis of biospecimens. In 2017, when President Barack Obama's administration had the opportunity to update the rules, they dropped the provisions that had been proposed to avoid what happened to Henrietta Lacks in the future—so currently, federally funded scientists still do not need to get permission from patients before using their cells, blood, tissue, or DNA for research.

An extreme form of unethical, unconsented medical practice takes place in developing countries whose hospitals are advanced enough to offer "Tourist Transplant" services. India, Pakistan, the Philippines, Egypt, and China, among other countries, have all been implicated. A report published in 2016[38] found a large discrepancy between official transplant figures from the Chinese government and the number of transplants reported by hospitals. While the government says 10,000 transplants occur each year, hospital data shows between 60,000 to 100,000 organs are transplanted each year. The report provides evidence that this gap is being made up by executed prisoners of conscience.

SKELETONS IN THE CLOSET:
HUMAN ZOOS AND IMPERIAL COLLECTIONS

Individuals and states have historically commoditized flora, fauna, and people. National interest in plants is fueled by agricultural relevance, while caged and displayed animals gave the public entertainment as well as

---

[38] "New Investigative Report: Exposing China's Lucrative Organ Transplant Industry." https://endtransplantabuse.org/an-update/.

evidence of Imperial success. Ethnological exhibits of human anatomical curiosities are common and were historically intended to objectify and stereotype indigenous peoples as brutish, uncivilized, and incapable of religion, for the purpose of further subjugation.

Science and slavery are deeply intertwined. James Petiver, one of the most important scientific figures many people have never heard of, ran a global network in the 1700s from London. Dozens of ship surgeons and captains collected animal and plant specimens for him in outlying colonies. Many of Petiver's collectors worked in the slave trade, largely because he and they had no other options: few ships outside the slave trade traveled to key points in Africa and Latin America. Petiver eventually amassed the largest natural history collection in the world, and it never would have happened without slavery.

While botany and entomology seem to have benefited the most from exotic ports of call such as Cartagena and Sierra Leone, a few physical sciences also piggybacked on the slave trade as well. Slave labor built the first major observatory in the Southern Hemisphere in Cape Town, South Africa. Astronomer Edmond Halley solicited observations of the moon and stars from slave ports, and geologists collected rocks and minerals there. When developing his theory of gravity, Isaac Newton needed tide readings from all over the globe to study the gravitational tug of the moon, and one crucial set of readings came from French slave ports in Martinique.

Thousands of specimens collected through the slave trade still reside in places such as the Natural History Museum in London, and are used to study plant domestication, historic climate change, and shifts in geographical distributions of species. Scientists have even extracted DNA from specimens to study how plants and animals have evolved across the centuries.

Scientific research not only depended on colonial slavery but enabled it and helped expand its reach. Quinine and other drugs helped Europeans survive in tropical locales.

Plants and animals are not the only vestiges of the transatlantic slave trade on display and in museums all over the world. From the mid-1800s to the late 20th century, indigenous and African people were kidnapped, enslaved, and exhibited in zoos under the guise of cultural anthropology or as a commodity available for colonial advantage.

Between 1878 and 1900, three groups of natives belonging to indigenous groups of Tehuelche, Selknam, and Kawésqar were shipped to Europe where they were treated and cared for poorly and expected to perform up to eight times per day in Human Zoos.[39] They were photographed, measured, weighed abroad, and hunted and murdered by Spanish conquistadors at home.

In the US, the vast majority, perhaps as much as 90 percent,[40] of all human remains curated by natural history museums are Native American. Adding to this are a smaller (but still significant) number of skeletons from African Americans, European Americans, and indigenous peoples originating from places all around the globe. Our fascination with the human body, and our propensity to buy, steal, or enslave humans and then turn them into trophies, scientific specimens, and valuable collectables, reflects a fundamentally racist worldview that does not see indigenous peoples as fully human. One such story exemplifies the intersection of slavery, colonialism, patriarchy, feminism, sexuality and the exploitation and exoticization of the Black female body, that of Sarah Baartman, the facts and intentions of whom were not recorded well by history.

One account of the life and times of Saartjie (Sarah) Baartman, a member of the Khoekhoe tribe from South Africa, claims that after her family was killed by Dutch hunters for sport (undisputed fact) she became a servant in a Dutch household. Tricked (disputed [41]) into believing that an Englishman paid the bride price to become her husband, Sarah agreed to go with him to Europe in 1810 as his wife, where she was told she would become famous. Instead, she was displayed (disputed if this was against

---

[39] "Selknam natives en route to Europe for being exhibited as animals in Human Zoos, 1899," Rare Historical Photos, December 2013. https://rarehistoricalphotos.com/selknam-natives-en-route-europe-exhibited-animals-human-zoos-1899/

[40] Redman, Samuel J., "How Many Human Skeletons Are in U.S. Museums?" History News Network, March 2016. https://historynewsnetwork.org/article/161946

[41] Dunton, Chris. "Sara Baartman and the Ethics of Representation" Research in African Literatures
Vol. 46, No. 2 (Summer 2015), pp. 32-51 (20 pages)
https://www.jstor.org/stable/10.2979/reseafrilite.46.2.32?seq=1

her will or her choice as a shrewd businesswoman) virtually naked at freak shows where members of her European audience often insulted and spat upon her. She was known as the Hottentot Venus (pejorative). The fascination with her naked body stems from a genetic variation called steatopygia, which leads to impressive accumulations of adipose tissue in the buttock region.

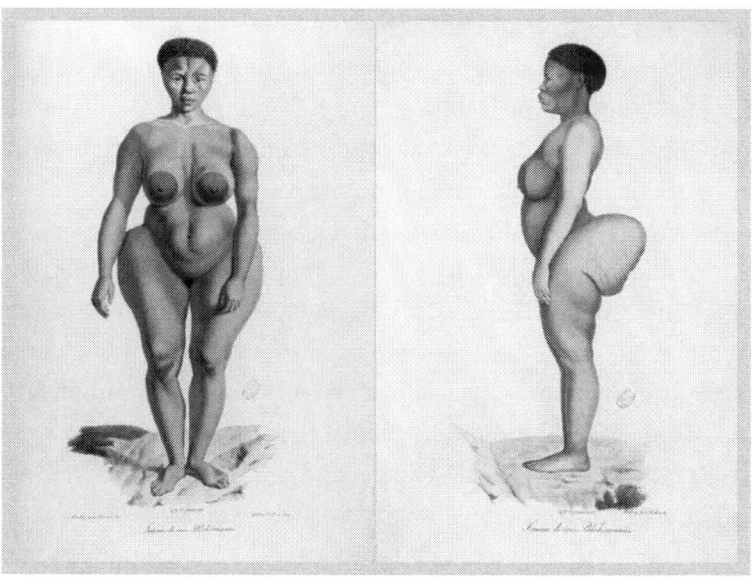

Image Credit: Wikimedia Commons.
https://commons.wikimedia.org/w/index.php?title=Special:Search&search=saartjie+ba
artman&fulltext=1&ns0=1&ns6=1&ns12=1&ns14=1&ns100=1&ns106=1#/media
/File:Sawtche_(dite_Sarah_Saartjie_Baartman),_%C3%A9tudi%C3%A9e_comm
e_Femme_de_race_B%C3%B4chismann,_Histoire_Naturelle_des_Mammif%C3
%A8res,_tome_II,_Cuvier,_Werner,_de_Lasteyrie.jpg.

Figure 2. Sarah "Saartjie" Baartman in Europe (ca.1790 - 1815), called the Hottentot Venus.

Four years after her arrival in London, she was moved to Paris, probably sold, where she fell under the control of a "showman of wild animals" at a travelling circus. When she was not being paraded for the masses, Baartman was displayed at society functions. It was at a ball for France's new establishment, where she arrived dressed in nothing but a few feathers, that Napoleon's surgeon general, Jean Léopold Nicolas Frédéric, Baron Cuvier, known as Georges Cuvier, a French naturalist and zoologist, sometimes referred to as the "founding father of paleontology," spotted her and claimed a scientific interest.

Over the following year she was repeatedly studied by doctors and anthropologists, who concluded that she was evidence of the superiority of the white race. Baartman lived in poverty and died in Paris of an undetermined inflammatory disease in December 1815. After her death, Cuvier dissected her body and displayed her remains. For more than a century and a half, visitors to the Museum of Man in Paris could view her brain, skeleton, and genitalia as well as a plaster cast of her body. Her remains were on public display until shame caught up with the administrators in 1976 and were returned to South Africa in 2002, and she was buried in the Eastern Cape on South Africa's National Women's Day.

Americans have had the right to bequeath their bodies to science since 1965, when the Uniform Anatomical Gift Act established the human body as property. With that law, a donor's wishes supersede those of the next of kin. This topic is explored further in relation to reproduction, where I look at the cases of "posthumous reproduction"; when a child tragically dies, do the parents have the right to retrieve their sperm and make offspring grandchildren from it?

Not only were live humans and human remains such as skeletons and casts, objects of entertainment but the performance of human autopsies (really dissections) were as well. Autopsy as a form of entertainment is a macabre concept, but in 1835 it helped to launch P. T. Barnum's career as the "Greatest Showman." A public and carefully orchestrated autopsy was staged in the amphitheater of the City Saloon on Broadway in New York City, where amidst 1,500 spectators, who each paid fifty cents for admission, anatomist Dr. David L. Rogers publicly dissected Joice Heth,[42] an African American slave that Barnum "leased" and publicly exhibited

---

[42] Wright, James R., "How the Public Autopsy of a Slave Joice Heth Launched P.T. Barnum's Career as the Greatest Showman on Earth," Clinical Anatomy 31: 956-965 (2018). https://dl.uswr.ac.ir/bitstream/Hannan/47891/1/2018%20ClinicalAnatomy%20Volume%2031%20Issue%207%20October%20%2820%29.pdf.

until her death. It was claimed that Heth was the 161-year-old nursemaid of George Washington, but her public dissection was meant to settle this question, and it was determined she could not have been more than 80 years old.

Live autopsies were not the only sideshow entertainment focused on humans. If you were a visitor to Coney Island in the early 20th century, aside from ethnographic exhibits similar to those mentioned above, you would be able to see the world's first premature infant incubator facility which claimed, "All The World Loves A Baby." Inside Martin Couney's Infant Incubator facility, the public paid 25 cents to view premature babies fighting for their lives. As the years passed, Couney's actual track record of saving premature infant lives developed the medical skills, knowledge, and technology that made premature infant medicine mainstream through this unusual avenue.

The gruesome and ghastly tradition of displaying the bodies of people without their consent, for public entertainment, continues to the modern era, and so does the sideshow element of medicine as entertainment. On one side of the coin, the Premier Exhibitions "Bodies Revealed" exhibit could not independently verify that the human remains were not those of persons incarcerated (likely victims of state-sanctioned torture or execution) in Chinese prisons. On the other side of the coin, social media challenges like the "Ice Bucket" challenge, although initially derided for the unusual avenue of raising funding for ALS research, generated $115 million dollars, dramatically accelerating the pace of discovery, with discovery of 5 new genes attributed directly to the Ice Bucket Challenge.[43]

---

[43] "Ice Bucket Challenge dramatically accelerated the fight against ALS." June 2019. https://www.als.org/stories-news/ice-bucket-challenge-dramatically-accelerated-fight-against-als

Chapter 2

BIRTH CONTROL

EUGENICS AND ETHICAL LAPSES IN THE QUEST FOR HORMONAL BIRTH CONTROL

On March 3, 1873, the US Congress passed federal regulations known as the Comstock Act. The statute defined contraceptives and information about sex and reproduction as obscene and illicit, making it a federal offense to disseminate birth control or even basic knowledge of menstrual cycles through the mail or across state lines.

The right of women to control their own reproduction—when and where to have a child—has been repressed for thousands of years. Margaret Sanger was born six years after the Comstock Acts were passed, into a desperately poor family with many children. She saw firsthand the effects of poverty, sickness, and hunger that having a large and unplanned family caused. She worked as an activist for social change her whole life so that every child born could be wanted and loved, and every woman in charge of her own destiny. She was the founder of Planned Parenthood and the scientist credited with spearheading the development of contemporary safe, effective, and affordable oral birth control pills and other hormonal methods, as well as securing the legal right of women to use such treatments.⁴⁴

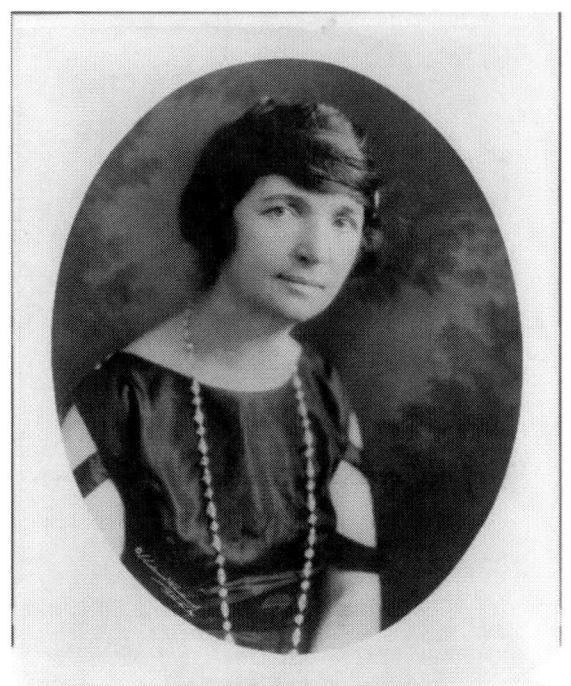

Image Source: Wikimedia Commons.
https://commons.wikimedia.org/w/index.php?search=margaret+Sanger&title=Special: Search&profile=advanced&fulltext=1&advancedSearch-current=%7B%7D&ns0=1&ns6=1&ns12=1&ns14=1&ns100=1&ns106=1#/media /File:Margaret_Sanger_LCCN2004672785.tif.

Figure 3. Margaret Sanger, Founder of Planned Parenthood.

However, she is a complex character in the history of reproduction, and similarly to J. Marion Sims (Chapter 1) her motivations, actions, and beliefs have been examined with respect to current mores and values and found to be abhorrent. She aligned with current theories of the day regarding eugenics—the "science" of improving society through planned

---

⁴⁴ "Margaret Sanger-Our Founder" by Planned Parenthood https://www.plannedparenthood.org/files/9214/7612/8734/Sanger_Fact_Sheet_Oct_2016.pdf.

breeding. Sanger's relationship with the eugenics movement was nuanced, she believed sterilization must be voluntary, and she did not align with malicious sterilization of whole races or religions. Sanger did, however, endorse the 1927 *Buck v. Bell* decision, written by Oliver Wendell Holmes, Jr., in which the Supreme Court ruled that compulsory sterilization of the "unfit" was allowable under the constitution.

Additionally, running counter to our modern theory of medical consent, the clinical trials for the birth control pill did not take place in the mainland United States, but in Puerto Rico, where poor women were given a strong formulation of the drug without being given "informed consent"; they were not told they were taking part in a trial or about any of the risks they may face. Three women died during this testing phase, but their deaths were never investigated[45].

On May 9, 1960, the US Food and Drug Administration (FDA) approved the sale of the first oral steroid birth control pills, only to married women for contraception, today more than 100 million women use the pill.

GRISWOLD VS. CONNECTICUT **(1965)**

New England residents lived under the most restrictive "Comstock" laws in the country. In Massachusetts, anyone disseminating contraceptives—or information about contraceptives—faced stiff fines and imprisonment. But by far the most restrictive state of all was Connecticut, where the act of using birth control was even prohibited by law. Married couples could be arrested for using birth control in the privacy of their own bedrooms and subjected to a one-year prison sentence. Prior to 1965, it was illegal in Connecticut to use any drug or device that prohibited contraception. Doctors across the entire country were prohibited from educating women about their reproductive health. Even explaining how the menstrual cycle worked could land a physician in jail, because women

---

[45] "Margaret Sanger-Our Founder" by Planned Parenthood https://www.plannedparenthood.org/files/9214/7612/8734/Sanger_Fact_Sheet_Oct_2016.pdf.

could take that knowledge and refrain from intercourse around the time of ovulation, preventing unwanted pregnancies. Several times, the Connecticut law was challenged, but it wasn't until 1965 when Estelle Griswold purposely opened a birth control clinic in New Haven, Connecticut, to get herself arrested in order to have "standing" to challenge the law.

In *Griswold v. Connecticut* (1965), the Supreme Court ruled that a state's ban on the use of contraceptives violated the right to marital privacy. After the dust settled surrounding *Griswold v. Connecticut*, it was still only legal for *married* women to have access to reproductive information, as the law was overturned on the grounds that the right to "marital privacy" was violated. It was not until 1972 that "The Pill" (the common nomenclature for the birth control pill) became available to all women regardless of marital status.

THE COLORADO EXPERIMENT

Barriers to contraceptive access are one reason for inconsistent or nonuse of contraception. Several innovative programs have been tested to increase access to various birth control methods. The aims of such programs are to reduce unwanted pregnancies, increase access by reducing the out-of-pocket costs to patients, increase awareness of different methods and education for use, and decrease costs for other State programs that address the effects of unwanted pregnancies (for example, labor and birth costs, housing, other social and emotional programs).

In the US there is a lot of misinformation about the safety of the hormonal birth control pill and it is not available over the counter.[46] Some of the misinformation is purposely spread through abstinence-only sex education programs for school-aged children. Students (and everyone!)

---

[46] Nelson AL, Rezvan A. A pilot study of women's knowledge of pregnancy health risks: implications for contraception. Contraception. 2012 Jan;85(1):78-82. doi: 10.1016/j.contraception.2011.04.011. Epub 2011 Jun 8. PMID: 22067804. https://pubmed.ncbi.nlm.nih.gov/22067804/.

need sexual education that's comprehensive, medically accurate, and free from shame and ideology. Abstinence-only sexual education programs have composed false information about all forms of contraception, yet a 2004 congressional report found that 80% of abstinence only programs give "false, misleading, or distorted" information about contraception.[47] In some cases, US federal grants have been obtained by antiabortion groups, and they have used the money to develop mobile technology (the FEMM smartphone app[48]) to sow doubts about the safety and effectiveness of the pill. This app is ineffective at preventing pregnancy, it collects very sensitive information, and has been downloaded more than 400,000 times.[49]

Women in over 80 countries[50] can already buy birth control pills without a prescription, including women just across the US border in Mexico. As medications go, the pill is very safe: safer than having a baby, driving, smoking, or taking daily aspirin. That said, the pill does have risks for women with medical conditions, including those with; blood clots, migraines, strokes, and certain cancers.

From 2009 to 2016, the state of Colorado spent $28 million supplying contraceptive intrauterine devices (IUDs) to 75 public health clinics throughout the state, several of which were based inside high schools. The program provided 43,713 contraceptive implants to women, plus trained medical staff on how to insert the devices. Colorado law allows those under 18 to give their own consent regarding birth control and sexual health services.

---

[47] More than 80 percent of the abstinence-only-until-marriage curricula reviewed contain false, misleading, or distorted information about reproductive health. The curricula reviewed misrepresent the effectiveness of contraceptives in preventing STDs and unintended pregnancy. They also contain false information about the risks of abortion, blur religion and science, promote gender stereotypes, and contain basic scientific errors. "The Content of Federally Funded Abstinence-Only Education Programs," Prepared for Rep. Henry A. Waxman, United States House of Representatives, Committee on Government Reform – Minority Staff, Special Investigations Division, December 2004.

[48] https://femmhealth.org/.

[49] Glenza, Jessica, "Anti-abortion group uses US federal grants to push controversial fertility app." The Guardian. July 29, 2019. https://www.theguardian.com/society/2019/jul/29/us-federal-grants-femm-app-natural-birth-control.

[50] Global Oral Contraception Availability. http://ocsotc.org/wp-content/uploads/worldmap/worldmap.html.

An analysis by University of Colorado researchers found the state program was responsible for as much as two-thirds of the decline in births to teen mothers from 2009 to 2015. The drop in pregnancies "averted" $66 million to $69.6 million that might have been spent on state and federal welfare and health care programs for low-income mothers, the researchers found.[51]

Plan B is an emergency contraception that can be used to prevent pregnancy if taken within 72 hours after unprotected sex. In 2012, Shippensburg University, a small Pennsylvania college, made national headlines for putting packs of Plan B in a vending machine in their student health center.

The roots of modern emergency contraception can actually be traced back to animal studies in the 1920s, yet human use started in the 1960s.

In the United States, the history of emergency contraception has sparked controversy, ignited political debates, and generated lawsuits. The heated nature of emergency contraception is due, in part, to whether or not people believe that the morning-after pill acts to prevent a pregnancy from occurring or whether it terminates a pregnancy that has already been established.

When birth control is restricted or access to it is denied it often impacts low-income communities, disenfranchised individuals, and women of color disproportionately.

One study from 2011 looked at what happened when the Catholic Loyola University Medical Center restricted access to injectable contraception for patients who had just given birth.[52] Pregnancy rates over the ensuing year increased, particularly for young women of color.

A 2005 study, for example, found that 54.9 percent of Catholic hospitals do not provide emergency contraception for any reason,

---

[51] Colorado Department of Public Health and Environment, Taking the Unintended Out of Pregnancy: Colorado's Success with Long-Acting Reversible Contraception, January 2017. http://www.colorado.gov/cdphe/cfpi-report.
[52] Guiahi M, McNulty M, Garbe G, Edwards S, Kenton K. "Changing depot medroxyprogesterone acetate access at a faith-based institution." *Contraception*. 2011 Sep;84(3):280-4. doi: 10.1016/j.contraception.2010.12.003. Epub 2011 Feb 2. PMID: 21843694. https://pubmed.ncbi.nlm.nih.gov/21843694/.

compared with 42.2% of non-Catholic hospitals. But another from 1999 found 82 percent of Catholic emergency departments do not provide emergency contraception, even for rape. Overall, women of color are more likely to give birth in Catholic institutions.

Seventy-five percent of incarcerated women are of reproductive age, most of whom are at-risk for unintended pregnancy. Women who are incarcerated come disproportionately from socioeconomically disadvantaged backgrounds and often lack access to reproductive health care. Although most state and federal prisons provide some level of care to prisoners, availability and access to medical care in jails varies considerably. For example, jail doctors in Salt Lake County, Utah, USA decide on a case-by-case basis who is given access to contraception.

Table 1. Timeline: Brief History of Emergency Contraception in the US[53]

Mid-1960s	Emergency contraception was used as a treatment for rape victims to prevent unintended pregnancy.
Late 1970s	Doctors began to offer the copper IUD as the only non-hormonal method of emergency contraception.
September 2, 1998	The Preven Emergency Contraception Kit became the first FDA-approved product specifically for emergency contraception.
July 28, 1999	The FDA-approved Plan B as the first progestin-only method of emergency contraception available in the US.
August 24, 2006	The FDA announced its approval of the sale of Plan B OTC to those age 18 and older whereas those younger than 18 would still need a prescription
September 2009	Plan B One-Step becomes available at retail pharmacies nationwide, and production of the old Plan B stops.
June 20, 2013	The FDA approves Plan B One-Step for over-the-counter sales with no age restrictions.

In fact, in 1976, the Hyde Amendment prohibited the use of federal funds for abortions, meaning federal prisons cannot provide abortion care. Women in immigration detention centers also face similar challenges in obtaining abortions, while at the same time experiencing increased rates of

---

[53] History of Plan B OTC. Princeton University. https://ec.princeton.edu/pills/planbhistory.html

hysterectomies that are not medically necessitated, explained, or appropriately consented.

The history of contraception includes significant victories and some defeats. In the end, the availability of this important contraceptive serves as one more tool in the prevention of unplanned pregnancies and abortions.

MEDICATION ABORTIONS AND ACCESS ON THE INTERNET

Since 2011, states have passed more than 400 restrictions[54] on abortion. As of 2017, 89 percent[55] of US counties had no abortion clinic, and about 40 percent of women of reproductive age live in one of those counties. As of the writing of this book, there are more than 20 states poised to outlaw abortion if given the opportunity, which would impact more than 25 million women of childbearing age. Extreme legislation that attempts to ban nearly all abortions, at all stages of pregnancy, with no exceptions in cases of rape or incest are being advanced in several states. In Alabama, the state senate passed the country's most restrictive abortion ban, with almost no exception at all possible (rape, incest, etc.). Its enactment has been delayed by challenges to it.

In many parts in the US, the rights conferred by *Roe v. Wade*— and reaffirmed in *Planned Parenthood v. Casey* and again in *Whole Woman's Health v. Hellerstedt*—have been significantly eroded. Women must travel hundreds of miles for in-state abortion access. They face up to 72-hour waiting periods, 20-week gestational bans, medically inaccurate informed consent materials—which include the false warning that abortion could be linked to breast cancer—restrictions on access to medication abortion, mandatory ultrasounds, and bans on insurance coverage for abortion.

---

[54] Jones, Rachel K., "As Danger to 'Roe' Grows, Many Voters May Not Even Know That Abortion Is Legal," Guttmacher Institute, September 2018. https://www.guttmacher.org/article/2018/09/danger-roe-grows-many-voters-may-not-even-know-abortion-legal.

[55] Jones RK, Witwer E, Jerman J, "Abortion Incidence and Service Availability in the United States, 2017," New York: Guttmacher Institute, 2019 https://www.guttmacher.org/report/abortion-incidence-service-availability-us-2017.

Other targeted restrictions on abortion providers (TRAP laws) have been enacted to allegedly protect the health and safety of women seeking abortion care but are medically useless, practically speaking. They mandate that abortion clinics be transformed into expensive, hospital-like surgical centers, as well as restrictions that attach to the abortion doctors themselves, like a requirement that abortionists have hospital-admitting privileges. Doctors don't get admitting privileges unless they regularly admit patients, however, abortion is one of the safest medical procedures[56] there is, so it is almost impossible for an abortion doctor to obtain admitting privileges.

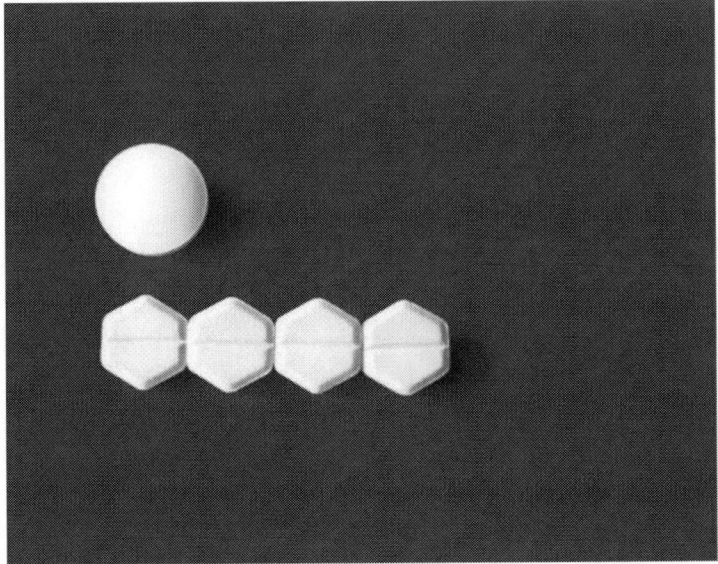

Image Source: Wikimedia Commons.
https://commons.wikimedia.org/wiki/File:Abortion_pill.jpg.

Figure 4. 200 mg mifepristone and 800 mcg misoprostol, the typical regimen for early medical abortion.

---

[56] Serious complications arising from aspiration abortions provided before 13 weeks are quite unusual. About 88% of the women who obtain abortions are less than 13 weeks pregnant. Of these women, 97% report no complications; 2.5% have minor complications that can be handled at the medical office or abortion facility; and less than 0.5% have more serious complications that require some additional surgical procedure and/or hospitalization. https://prochoice.org/wp-content/uploads/safety_of_abortion.pdf.

All of these restrictions, plus the accessibility of telehealth and digital pharmacies, have led to a phenomenon called "self-managed abortion," when a person chooses to have an abortion outside of a medical setting. The "abortion pill" (medication abortion) is a combination of mifepristone and misoprostol and can be purchased online and shipped directly to a prospective patient. Women on Web[57], a nonprofit organization that provides online information and access to abortion, has an online service that can connect visitors in highly restricted countries with a licensed doctor who can provide them with medication abortion. Some sites, like Plan C[58], connect people with medication abortion suppliers online for a cost ($90 to $430). Plan C also created a "report card" that grades online abortion pill retailers based on their pricing, shipping time, product quality, and physician oversight. Aid Access[59] is an online abortion pill retailer run by Dutch doctor Rebecca Gomperts. The site is currently the only abortion pill service operated by a licensed physician who counsels patients and writes the prescription for the pills. Patients send the prescription to Aid Access's overseas pharmacy, which ships the medication to the US.

Prosecutors are trying to criminalize self-managed abortions or even having a stillbirth child, and are using Internet searches, browsing history, and text messages to punish some women for ending their pregnancies. These cases overwhelmingly target women of color. According to the reproductive justice legal group If/When/How[60], there are five states—Arizona, Delaware, Idaho, Oklahoma, and South Carolina—that still have laws on the books criminalizing self-managed abortion.

Period Poverty

The cost of menstrual hygiene products amounts to a tax on those who have uteruses. Levied against the bodies of children, inmates, refugees, the

---

[57] https://www.womenonweb.org/.
[58] https://plancpills.org/.
[59] https://aidaccess.org/.
[60] https://www.ifwhenhow.org/.

homeless, and many other vulnerable groups every month for roughly 30 years, amounts to oppressive discrimination. As far as products made of paper and cotton go, why should they be taxed as luxury goods?? As a fundamental instrument of basic hygiene for over 50% of the population, the US Food and Drug Administration defines menstrual products as medical devices, others of which—diabetic test strips and insulin devices, for example—readily receive tax exemptions.

"Pink Tax" is a term used generally to mean the cost of any good or service for women that is higher than a similar good or service for men (think of almost anything—from haircuts to dry cleaning) and Tampon Tax is a term used specific to for the tax imposed on menstrual hygiene products by a government. These products are not subject to a unique or special tax in these jurisdictions but classified as luxury items along with other goods that are not exempted. As of November 2019, 34 state governments in the US levy sales tax on menstrual hygiene products, such as pads and tampons.[61]

Taxing them is unconstitutional and discriminates against those who need to use them. Governments can and do exempt products from consumption tax if they deem them important enough. Alternatively, they can tax them at a rate lower than other, non-essential items.

Kenya was the first country to abolish a tampon tax in 2004. Other countries that don't tax these goods as luxury items include Australia, Uganda, Canada, India, Nicaragua, Malaysia, and Lebanon. The UK tax rate will go to zero as of Jan. 1, 2021.

How much does this tax add up to on those uterus owners who experience menstruation?

In California alone, it has been estimated that removing taxes on feminine hygiene products would cost the state about $20 million, which is why it keeps getting voted down. New York State lost 14 million dollars the year it ends the tax.

---

[61] Phelan, Jessica. "Tampon tax is real. Women everywhere pay their governments extra to have periods." GlobalPost, August 2015. https://www.google.com/amp/s/www.pri.org/stories/2015-08-15/tampon-tax-real-women-everywhere-pay-their-governments-extra-have-periods%3famp.

The estimate for the whole United States? Between 4 and 9 percent.

Sales tax varies from state to state and of the 50 in the union, only five waive it on sanitary goods: Maryland, Massachusetts, Minnesota, New Jersey, and Pennsylvania. Five others don't have a sales tax. The rest do, and don't exempt tampons from it.

Dozens of states are now considering bills to require public schools to supply free tampons and other menstrual products in their bathrooms. Often youth led, the menstrual equity movement [62] seeks to make sure all students can afford or access menstrual supplies without shame or stigma, and with the goal of uninterrupted education.

Jails and prisons are another source of menstrual distress and poverty. Period products are expensive to purchase, but made out of the cheapest, flimsiest materials possible. Women and those who bleed, improvise, making do with sheets, clothes, toilet paper, and other materials. Menstrual products can be strictly rationed. There are reports of accidentally leaking menstrual blood on clothes, linens, and the floor—inciting punishment. In Kentucky, a judge had to stop a court proceeding because a female inmate had been denied menstrual products for 2-3 days and was wearing inappropriate and bloodied clothing to the court.[63]

In late 2020, Scotland became the first country in the world to allow free and universal access to menstrual products, including tampons and pads, in any public facilities, such as schools and universities.

---

[62] https://www.freethetampons.org/
[63] https://www.youtube.com/watch?v=RUKCIHzTR-0

Chapter 3

COITUS

CONTAGIOUS DISEASES ACT

When gonorrhea was recognized as an agent that can cause sterility in women by Emil Noeggerath in 1872,[64] this was a revolutionary idea. Louis Pastuer had just consolidated the controversial germ (microscopic organisms) theory of disease in 1860-1864. In 1879, Albert Neisser identified the gonococcus bacteria itself.

In 1864, obsessive fear of venereal disease led the Parliament of the United Kingdom to enact the Contagious Diseases Act, with the goal of preventing venereal diseases within the armed forces. The Contagious Diseases Act made women suspected of prostitution register with the police and submit to an invasive medical examination. This legislation essentially allowed for police officers to arrest women suspected of being prostitutes. If the woman was found to be suffering from a venereal disease, she would be confined to a "lock hospital" until pronounced "clean." The alternative to agreeing to the examination was three months imprisonment (extended to six months in the 1869 act) or hard labor. The acts did not enforce the examination of men.

---

[64] Noeggerath E. "Latent gonorrhea, especially with regard to its influence on fertility in women." *Am J Obstet Gynecol.* 1951;62(4):726–31.

34   *Carol Lynn Curchoe Burton*

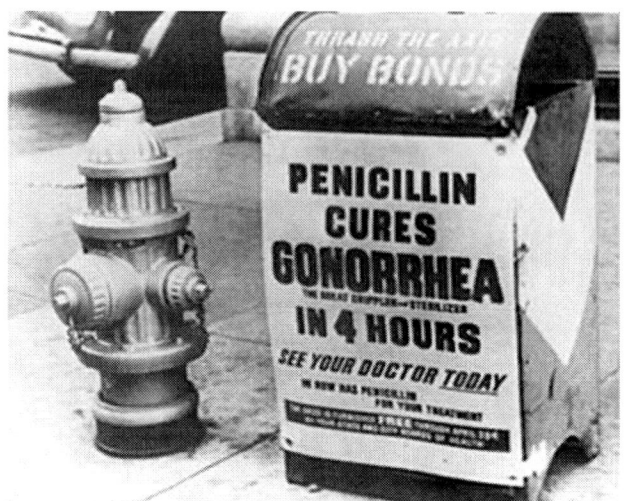

Image Source: Wikimedia Commons.
https://commons.wikimedia.org/wiki/File:Penicillin_cures_gonorrhea.jpg.

Figure 5. An advertisement for penicillin as a cure for gonorrhea (1940s in South Carolina).

PREMARITAL BLOOD TESTS

In the US, "vice reform" was infused into the progressive agenda of the early 1900s. Historically, many states[65] have required applicants for a marriage license to obtain a blood test. These tests were for venereal diseases (most commonly syphilis), for genetic disorders (such as sickle-cell anemia), or for rubella. The tests for syphilis were part of a broad public health campaign enacted in the late 1930s by US Surgeon General Thomas Parran.

Similar to many invasive procedures mandated by governments, mandatory blood tests for couples seeking marriage licenses were a

---

[65] By the end of 1938, twenty-six states had enacted provisions prohibiting the marriage of infected individuals.

product of the age of eugenics and Progressive politics.[66] As Ruth C. Engs notes in *The Progressive Era's Health Reform Movement*[67]: "Racial improvement" through positive eugenics, such as marriage to a healthy individual, [and] blood tests for syphilis prior to marriage ... were promoted for improving the 'race,' thus leading to a healthier nation."

Though Progressive reformers achieved many noteworthy goals during this period [68], they also promoted discriminatory policies and espoused intolerant ideas. The Wilson administration, for instance, despite its embrace of modernity and progress, pursued a racial agenda that culminated in the segregation of the federal government.

Today, only one state, Montana, continues to require blood tests.[69] Between 1980 and 2008, the remaining requirements for blood tests were abolished.

It is important to understand this historical context, as it continues to have implications today. Morally centered agendas influence the types of interventions that are funded relating to sexual health education for children, fertility education, reduction of blood borne disease risk (HIV and HepB among others) and among high-risk groups: injection drug users, men who have sex with men, and sex workers. However, harm reduction approaches have demonstrated much more success, including, peer

---

[66] The period of US history from the 1890s to the 1920s is usually referred to as the Progressive Era, an era of intense social and political reform aimed at making progress toward a better society.

[67] Religious, political, social, and health reform earmarked the Progressive Era. The era's health reform movement—like today's clean-living movement—saw campaigns against alcohol, tobacco, drugs, and sexuality. It included crusades for exercise, vegetarian diets, and alternative health care and concerns about eugenics and new diseases. Covering the years leading up to the Progressive Era through the 1920s, this book provides entries on the central figures, events, crusades, legislation, publications, and terms of the health reform movements, while a detailed timeline ties health reform to political, social, and religious movements. Eng, Ruth C., The Progressive Era's Health Reform Movement, Praeger Publishers, Westport, CT, 2003.

[68] McGerr, Michael. "A Fierce Discontent: The Rise and Fall of The Progressive Movement in America." Oxford University Press.

[69] Marriage License Requirements, FindLaw, October 2018. https://family.findlaw.com/marriage/marriage-license-requirements.html.

education[70], condom negotiating skills, safety tips, male and female condoms[71], prevention-care, and more.

MARRIAGE ANNULMENT AND IMPOTENCE

Reproduction has historically been a central tenet of the marriage contract. Infertility and surrogacy are mentioned in the Old Testament, including when Sarah was unable to have children in her old age, prompting her to ask Abraham to sleep with Hagar, an Egyptian slave.

Researchers have discovered ancient (4,000-year-old) evidence of surrogacy[72] while studying an Assyrian clay tablet that contains the oldest known marriage contract with language on infertility and surrogacy. The contract details how a man named Laqipum and his bride, Hatala, will move forward with surrogacy if they don't have a child within two years.

As with divorce, a decree of annulment ends a marriage. But, unlike with divorce, a decree of annulment declares that no valid marriage ever existed because of some defect at its inception. Compared with divorce, annulments have always been relatively rare, although they often appeal to devout Roman Catholics who, if a first marriage is annulled, can then remarry without objection from the Church. Annulments are, in theory, tightly regulated. Each state provides specific circumstances in which a marriage can be annulled. Typical grounds for annulment include bigamy, impotence, infancy, mental incompetence, incest, fraud, and duress—all

---

[70] Gollub, Erica L et al. "Three city feasibility study of a body empowerment and HIV prevention intervention among women with drug use histories: Women FIT." *Journal of women's health* (2002) vol. 19,9 (2010): 1705-13. doi:10.1089/jwh.2009.1778. https://www.ncbi.nlm.nih.gov/pmc/articles/PMC2953934/

[71] Campbell, Aimee N C et al. "Female condom skill and attitude: results from a NIDA Clinical Trials Network gender-specific HIV risk reduction study." AIDS education and prevention : official publication of the International Society for AIDS Education vol. 23,4 (2011): 329-40. doi:10.1521/aeap.2011.23.4.329 https://www.ncbi.nlm.nih.gov/pmc/articles/PMC3162343/

[72] Ahmet Berkiz Turp, Ismail Guler, Nuray Bozkurt, Aysel Uysal, Bulent Yilmaz, Mustafa Demir & Onur Karabacak (2018) Infertility and surrogacy first mentioned on a 4000-year-old Assyrian clay tablet of marriage contract in Turkey, Gynecological Endocrinology, 34:1, 25-27, DOI: 10.1080/09513590.2017.1391208 https://www.tandfonline.com/doi/abs/10.1080/09513590.2017.1391208?journalCode=igye20.

impediments to lawful marriage that must have existed at the time the union was celebrated to be valid grounds.

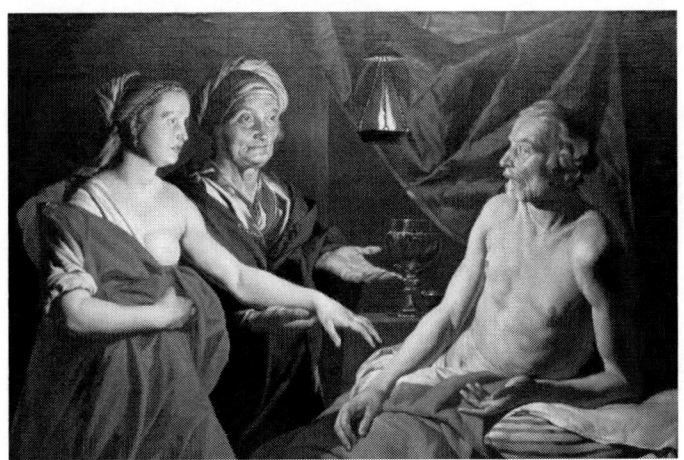

Image Source: Wikimedia Commons.
https://commons.wikimedia.org/wiki/File:1638_Stom_Sarah_fuehrt_Abraham_Hagar_zu_anagoria.JPG.

Figure 6. Sarah Leading Hagar to Abraham (Stom, Berlin).

The so-called "essentials of the marriage" test that was followed in most states dates to an 1862 Massachusetts case, *Reynolds v. Reynolds*. In that case, the court granted an annulment to Michael Reynolds, whose wife, Bridget, had passed herself off as "chaste and virtuous" while secretly being pregnant with another man's child. Had Bridget merely been "defiled and debauched," the court reasoned, Michael would have no right to an annulment because misrepresentations as to "character, fortune, health, or temper," or other "accidental qualities" would not be enough to make a marriage voidable. But Bridget's sin was greater, in the court's eyes, because it undermined her husband's implicit "right to require that his wife shall not bear to his bed aliens to his blood and lineage." Moreover, the court noted, as a pregnant woman, she was "incapable of bearing a child to her husband at the time of her marriage," and thus "unable to perform an important part of the contract." Her concealed pregnancy thus went to the "essentials of the marriage."

As it developed in most states, the "essentials of the marriage" test tended to restrict annulments based on fraud to those cases involving misrepresentations about sex or procreation, those matters that were fundamental to the very definition of marriage. Thus, plaintiffs who alleged that their spouses lied about pregnancy, infertility, impotence, frigidity, venereal disease, or their willingness to have children were more successful in obtaining annulments than those who complained of misrepresentations about wealth (fraud), character, or mental capacity.

Chapter 4

STERILIZATION

On November 8, 1895, at the University of Würzburg, Germany, the physicist Wilhelm Conrad Röntgen discovered a new, unknown type of ray, which he named X-rays. X-rays soon became a funfair attraction. People stood in long lines, for a chance to see their bodies in X-ray light. Shoe-fitting fluoroscopes, sold under the names X-ray Shoe Fitter, Pedoscope, and Foot-o-scope, were X-ray fluoroscope machines installed in shoe stores from the 1920s until about the 1970s in the United States, Canada, United Kingdom, South Africa, Germany, and Switzerland as a sales gimmick to sell shoes to children. The long-term effects of radiation-induced cancer was unknown. Children, we now know, are twice as sensitive to radiation than adults.[73]

As X-rays began to be used more frequently for medical applications, the sterilizing effects of X-rays when applied to human ovaries and testicles were noted as early as 1903.

Covering the testicles and ovaries during X-rays has been recommended since the 1950s, when studies in fruit flies prompted concern that radiation might damage human DNA and cause birth defects.

---

[73] Little JB (2000). "Chapter 14: Ionizing Radiation." In Kufe DW, Pollock RE, Weichselbaum RR, Bast RC Jr, Gansler TS, Holland JF, Frei E III (eds.). Cancer medicine (6th ed.). Hamilton, Ont: B.C. Decker. ISBN 1-55009-113-1.

At least 46 states require shielding of reproductive organs if they are close to the area being examined, unless shielding would interfere with the diagnostic quality of the exam, according to The American Association of Physicists in Medicine.[74] Fear of radiation is embedded in our subconscious. However, in the past decade radiology professionals have started to reassess the practice of draping, based on changes in imaging technology and a better understanding of radiation's effects. It seems shielding doesn't protect against the greatest radiation effect: "scatter," which occurs when radiation ricochets inside the body, including under the shield, and eventually deposits its energy in tissues. Several groups have recommended shielding of patients be "discontinued as routine practice," including the American College of Radiology and the Image Gently Alliance, which promotes safe pediatric imaging.[75]

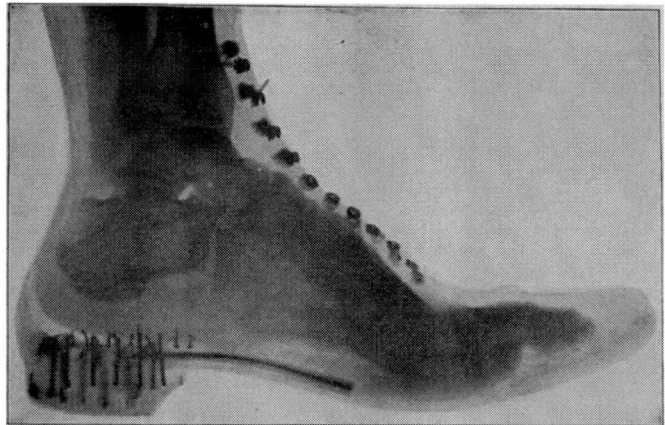

Image source: Wikimedia Commons.
https://commons.wikimedia.org/wiki/File:American_X-ray_journal_(1902)_
 (14777271093).jpg.

Figure 7. American X-ray journal (1902) Shoe Fitting Fluoroscope.

---

[74] American Association of Physicists in Medicine. https://www.aapm.org/
[75] Jaklevic, Mary Chris, "No Shield From X-rays: How Science Is Rethinking Lead Aprons," KHN, January 2020. https://khn.org/news/no-shield-from-x-rays-how-science-is-rethinking-lead-aprons/

EUGENIC STERILIZATION

Forcing a woman to terminate a pregnancy she wants or to continue a pregnancy that she does not want both violate the same human rights: the right to decide freely whether and when to bear a child and the right to have that decision respected by the government.

In the latter half of the 20th century, attention to reproductive rights violations has focused largely on actions by governments to curtail what they view as "overpopulation."

In India in the 1970s, the national government was concerned about the impact of high population growth rates on deepening poverty. They established population targets, condoned mandatory sterilization laws among various Indian states, and designed punitive disincentives for large families, resulting in a dark era of widespread coercion and reproductive abuses.

In the 1990s, under former President Alberto Fujimori's regime, Peru sanctioned coercive and forced sterilizations of more than 346,000 poor and indigenous women and almost 25,000 men through intimidation and force.[76]

The first eugenics law in the United States was passed in Connecticut in 1895, and it was a law against certain kinds of marriages. However, it was ineffective at stopping reproduction among these groups, so policy makers turned to a philosophy of "segregation" to institutionalize certain people deemed "unfit" for their reproductive years. Segregation was quite an expensive proposition, so eugenic sterilization followed.

In 1927, the US Supreme Court decided, by a vote of 8 to 1, to uphold a state's right to forcibly sterilize a person considered unfit to procreate. The case, known as *Buck v. Bell*, centered on a young woman named Carrie Buck, whom the state of Virginia had deemed to be "feebleminded." As many as 70,000 Americans were forcibly sterilized during the 20th century.

---

[76] Cabitza M, "Peru women fight for justice over forced sterilization," BBC News, Dec. 6, 2011, http://www.bbc.co.uk/news/world-latin-america-15891372.

The Family Planning Services and Public Research Act of 1970, often called Title X Family Planning Program, is a US federal law that provides federal funding for family planning services to low income or uninsured families. The US federal government passed the law, Public Law 91-572, in 1970 as an amendment to the Public Health Services Act of 1944. The Act created the Office of Population Affairs (OPA) under the Secretary of Health, Education, and Welfare (here called the Secretary). Through the Act, the OPA and the Secretary provide resources and policy advice to the US government on health issues. The OPA also issued grants and formed contracts with public and nonprofit organizations to assist in the establishment and operation of voluntary family planning services. The Act helped to extend reproductive health services to low-income individuals and to individuals who otherwise struggle to get such services.

Title X provided those in the US, especially those in lower socioeconomic classes, with access to birth control and education about birth control. As a result of Title X, the federal government regulated all clinics receiving Title X funds. Clinics that received Title X funds were required to follow uniform regulations and guidelines that guarantee women access to contraceptive counseling, a range of contraception options, confidentiality of services, and referral for other health and social services when necessary.

After the Family Planning Services and Population Research Act of 1970, physicians sterilized perhaps 25% of Native American women of childbearing age, and there is evidence suggesting that the numbers were actually higher. Some of these procedures were performed under pressure or duress, or without the women's knowledge or understanding. The law subsidized sterilizations for patients who received their health care through the Indian Health Service and for Medicaid patients, and Black and Latina women were also targets of coercive sterilization in these years. By the end of the decade, advocacy by Native women and other women of color resulted in the adoption of federal regulations that offered women some protections from unwanted sterilization procedures. The new regulations required, for example, an extended waiting period, from 72 hours to 30 days, between consent and an operation.

CHEMICAL AND SURGICAL CASTRATION

The first reported attempt of hormonal manipulation to reduce pathological sexual behavior occurred in 1944, when diethylstilbestrol was prescribed to lower testosterone levels.[77] Medroxyprogesterone acetate and cyproterone acetate have been used throughout the United States, Canada, and some European countries to diminish sexual fantasies and sexual impulses in sexual offenders. Chemical castration has been executed without informed consent in Korea and in three states of the United States.[78]

In July 2011, Korea introduced the concept of chemical castration of sexual offenders. Under the current law, perpetrators of sexual crimes against minors aged less than 16 years are subject to chemical castration. In 1996, California became the first state in the United States to authorize the use of either chemical or surgical castration for certain sexual offenders who were being released from prison. It is now one of eight states that allow chemical or surgical castration of sex offenders. They are California, Florida, Georgia, Louisiana, Montana, Oregon, Texas, and Wisconsin. In 1996, California became the first state in the United States to authorize the use of either chemical or surgical castration for certain sexual offenders who were being released from prison. It is now one of eight states that allow chemical or surgical castration of sex offenders, as a condition of release from custody. They are: California, Florida, Georgia, Louisiana, Montana, Oregon, Texas, and Wisconsin. Medroxyprogesterone acetate (MPA) treatment or its equivalent is the common method of chemical castration. MPA, an artificial female hormone, (commonly sold under the name Depo-Provera), when used by men, MPA has the effect of reducing their testosterone levels to pre-puberty levels. Chemical castration using Luteinizing hormone-releasing hormone (LHRH) agonists reduces

---

[77] Miller RD. "Forced administration of sex-drive reducing medications to sex offenders: treatment or punishment?" *Psychol Public Policy Law*. 1998 Mar-Jun; 4(1-2):175-99.

[78] Scott CL, Holmberg T, J. "Castration of sex offenders: prisoners' rights versus public safety." *Am Acad Psychiatry Law*. 2003; 31(4):502-9.

circulating testosterone to very low levels, and results in very low levels of recidivism.[79]

In the United Kingdom, computer scientist Alan Turing, famous for his contributions to mathematics and computer science, pleaded guilty in 1952 to a charge of gross indecency for having a homosexual relationship and accepted chemical castration as a term of his probation, thus avoiding imprisonment. At the time, homosexual acts between males were illegal and homosexual orientation was widely considered to be a mental illness that could be treated with chemical castration. Turing experienced side effects such as gynecomastia (breast enlargement) and bloating of his physique.

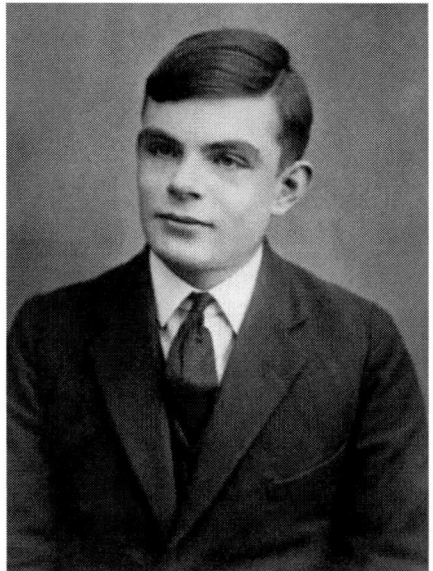

Image Source: Wikimedia Commons.
https://commons.wikimedia.org/wiki/File:Alan_Turing_Aged_16.jpg.

Figure 8. Alan Turing, Aged 16. English mathematician, computer scientist, logician, cryptanalyst, philosopher, and theoretical biologist. Turing is widely considered to be the father of theoretical computer science and artificial intelligence.

---

[79] Weinberger LE, Sreenivasan S, Garrick T, Osran H. "The impact of surgical castration on sexual recidivism risk among sexually violent predatory offenders." *J Am Acad Psychiatry Law*. 2005;33(1):16-36. PMID: 15809235. https://pubmed.ncbi.nlm.nih.gov/15809235/.

ACCESS TO ENDOMETRIUM ABLATION AND TUBAL LIGATIONS

According to the journal *Obstetrics & Gynecology*, female (or male) sterilization is the most common method of contraception in the United States,[80] with about 700,000 women undergoing the procedure per year. Yet, many doctors will not even broach the subject let alone perform the procedure on women under 30 years old. It is very common for doctors to deny tubal ligations to people with uteruses who don't have children or are "young" (a poorly defined metric!).[81] There is a sort of cultural belief that all women will want to have children, or that they don't "know their own minds," if they think they don't. Other reasons doctors might give are that maybe a future spouse might want kids, or they might regret it. Essentially, someone other than the person requesting the surgery knows better than they do. Reasons that people who have uteruses give, such as they have a partner who wants to carry pregnancies, already care for children, or may experience severe gender dysmorphia, are often swept under the rug. There are often long waiting periods[82] (up to 30 days and in many cases years of counseling) required.

Men, on the other hand, can walk into any clinic and procure a vasectomy in under five minutes without moral scrutiny or deterrents, without needing multiple appointments, no questioning, no stigma, and no shame.

---

[80] Bartz, Deborah, and James A Greenberg. "Sterilization in the United States." Reviews in obstetrics & gynecology vol. 1,1 (2008): 23-32. https://www.ncbi.nlm.nih.gov/pmc/articles/PMC2492586/.

[81] Date, S., Rokade, J., Mule, V., & Dandapannavar, S. (2014). "Female sterilization failure: Review over a decade and its clinicopathological correlation." *International Journal of Applied and Basic Medical Research,* 4(2), 81. doi: 10.4103/2229-516x.136781.

[82] Health care justice and its implications for current policy of a mandatory waiting period for elective tubal sterilization. Moaddab et. Al. conclude that Medicaid policy allocates access to elective tubal sterilization differently, based on source of payment and gender, which violates health care justice in both its deontologic and consequentialist dimensions. Obstetricians should invoke health care justice in women's health care as the basis for advocacy for needed change in law and health policy, to eliminate health care injustice in women's access to elective tubal sterilization. https://www.ajog.org/article/S0002-9378(15)00330-0/pdf.

The Vatican has recently clarified its opposition to hysterectomies,[83] saying it's OK to remove a uterus that is "no longer suitable for procreation."

The Vatican issued a statement, if "medical experts have reached the certainty" that any future pregnancy would end in a "spontaneous abortion" before viability, then the patient can have a hysterectomy, because it won't have the (immoral) effect of sterilizing them.

The Catholic Church opposes reproductive health care that interferes with procreation, including abortion, tubal ligations, vasectomies, and most contraception. In the United States, directives issued by the US Conference of Catholic Bishops govern one in six acute-care hospital beds; in some states the number is closer to half. In at least 46 regions nationwide, a Catholic hospital is the only accessible option.

---

[83] Harris, Elise. "Vatican't doctrine czar approves hysterectomies in 'extreme cases.'" Crux. January 2019. https://cruxnow.com/vatican/2019/01/vaticans-doctrine-czar-approves-hysterectomies-in-extreme-cases/

Chapter 5

PARTURITION

THE ROYAL ROOTS OF "BACK LABOR"

Childbirth is universal, but class, culture, ethnicity, and the scientific and political flux of medicine influence how women experience it, historically and now. The maternal birthing position has evolved over time. Modern maternal birthing positions are typically dorsal or lithotomy (supine position of the body with the legs separated, flexed, and supported in raised stirrups). Various explanations for the change in position from upright to horizontal have been proposed including facilitating use of forceps, promoting men's power over women (both midwives and parturients), and use of anesthesia, among others.

Some of the earliest records of labor show women in a sitting, squatting, or standing position while laboring. An ancient sculpture from Egypt shows Cleopatra (69–30BC) kneeling down to give birth, surrounded by five attendants. Evidence of birthing stools and chairs date back to Babylonian times.[84] Certainly, lying down is not considered to be the historical birthing position of choice. In a 1961 survey of 76 traditional

---

[84] Dundes, Lauren, "The Evolution of Maternal Birthing Position." *Public Health: Then and Now*, *American Journal of Public Health*, 1987. https://ajph.aphapublications.org/doi/pdf/10.2105/AJPH.77.5.636.

cultures, only 18 percent of women assumed either a prone or dorsal birthing position.[85]

King Louis XIV had 22 children over his lifespan (1638–1715). As a king, he had very good reasons to have many children, given that he needed a guaranteed heir to the throne. But he also apparently liked to watch his wives and mistresses pushing out his children. Louis "enjoyed watching women giving birth, he became frustrated by the obscured view of birth when it occurred on a birthing stool." Because of this he "promoted the new reclining position. He also insisted on male accoucheurs [midwives] attending births."

EPISIOTOMY AND INTERVENTIONS

Before the 1990s, childbirth it seems was "too common" to be highly traumatic. According to the World Health Organization, 803 women die from complications related to pregnancy and childbirth every day.[86] This doesn't take into account the life-changing injuries women can suffer during childbirth. A few studies estimate that 4% of births lead to postnatal PTSD. One study from 2003 found that around a third of mothers who experience a "traumatic delivery," defined as involving complications, the use of instruments to assist delivery or near death, go on to develop PTSD. Postnatal PTSD was only formally recognized in the US in the 1990s when the American Psychiatry Association changed its description of what constitutes a traumatic event from "something outside the range of usual human experience," to someone who "witnessed or confronted serious physical threat or injury to themselves or others."

In the US, mothers birthing at hospitals are hooked up to continuous electronic monitoring equipment to track the baby's heartbeat and identify

---

[85] Narroll, F et al. "Position of women in childbirth. A study in data quality control." *American journal of obstetrics and gynecology* vol. 82 (1961): 943-54. doi:10.1016/s0002-9378(16)36172-5. https://pubmed.ncbi.nlm.nih.gov/14478406/.

[86] "Maternal mortality." World Health Organization. September 2019. https://www.who.int/news-room/fact-sheets/detail/maternal-mortality.

possible signs of distress—even though continuous monitoring offers very little benefit for the majority of births and is actually associated with a higher rate of C-sections and vaginal deliveries with forceps.[87]

The most common reason that a recto-vaginal fistula occurs in the United States today is traumatic vaginal delivery.[88] The major risk factors for such injuries are forceps delivery with or without episiotomy, delivery with a vacuum extractor with or without episiotomy, shoulder dystocia, fetal distress (requiring prompt delivery to protect the life and health of the baby), and long labor (which is not the same as prolonged obstructed labor).

Before the common use of the Cesarean section, all babies had to be passed through the birth canal. Obviously, babies can become obstructed if they are breech or too large. This reality has led to untold horrors visited upon laboring women, throughout history until the present day, as delivery methods and instruments have been relentlessly sought. There is a modern day cultural war being waged between "natural birth" advocates and the current "standard of care," which often calls for over-monitoring and increased interventions, and yet somehow still leads to a horrific maternal fetal death rate in the US.[89]

The history of traumatic interventions starts with episiotomy (an incision made in the perineum — the tissue between the vaginal opening and the anus) surgery, the progenitor of which was the "symphysiotomy," an obstetric procedure first used in 1597 for quickly removing a child from a woman's womb—and used for almost three centuries thereafter. The procedure involves dividing the cartilage of the pubic symphysis to widen the pelvis, allowing childbirth when there is a "mechanical" problem. In

---

[87] Alfirevic, Z et al. "Continuous cardiotocography (CTG) as a form of electronic fetal monitoring (EFM) for fetal assessment during labour." *The Cochrane database of systematic reviews* ,3 CD006066. 19 Jul. 2006, doi:10.1002/14651858.CD006066. https://pubmed.ncbi.nlm.nih.gov/16856111/.

[88] "Vaginal Fistulas." Mount Sinai. https://www.mountsinai.org/care/obgyn/services/fistula-care.

[89] Women in the US had the highest rate of maternal mortality because of complications from pregnancy or childbirth; women in Sweden and Norway had among the lowest rates. High rates of Cesarean sections, lack of prenatal care, and increased rates of obesity, diabetes, and heart disease may be contributing factors to the high rate in the US. https://www.commonwealthfund.org/publications/issue-briefs/2018/dec/womens-health-us-compared-ten-other-countries.

some cases, sections of pelvic bone were also removed. The procedure was originally performed by hand using a small knife and saw to remove the bone, without anesthesia to a woman in the middle of giving birth. It took a long time, and it was messy and obviously painful, therefore two intrepid doctors invented the precursor to the modern chainsaw in 1780 to make the removal of pelvic bone easier and less time-consuming and more accurate. The symphysiotomy tool was powered by a hand crank and looked like a modern-day kitchen knife with little teeth on a chain.

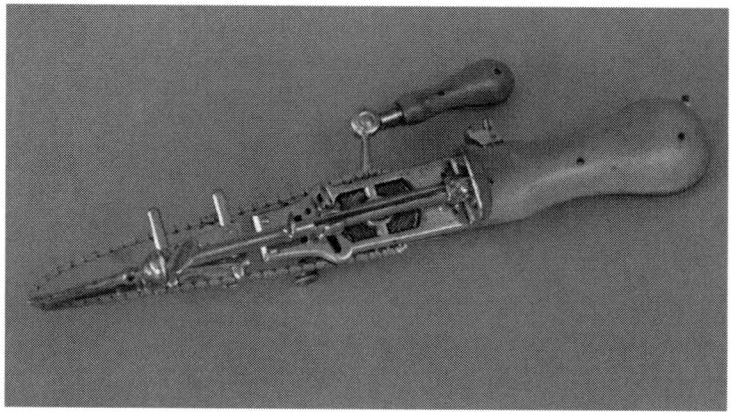

Image Source: Wikimedia Commons.
https://en.wikipedia.org/wiki/Chainsaw#/media/File:Osteotome3.jpg.

Figure 9. Historical osteotome, a medical bone chainsaw.

Symphysiotomy is a controversial operation that was seldom used after the mid-20th century, but which was carried out on an estimated 1,500 women without their consent in Ireland between the 1940s and 1980s. As Cesarean sections grew safer, the use of the operation declined. The master of Dublin's National Maternity Hospital (NMH), Alex Spain, disapproved of C-sections for religious reasons. Jacqueline Morrissey, a historian who began investigating the practice in the 1990s, believes it was Spain's Catholic beliefs that caused him to shun Cesarean sections. At the time, it was thought that having multiple Cesarean sections was dangerous, and that further pregnancies would have to be stopped by sterilization or contraception. Marie O'Connor, the chair of Survivors of Symphysiotomy, also notes that the practice was driven by the need to train students so that the surgery, which did not require electricity, could be carried out in rural parts of Africa and other "low resource" settings. These operations were performed without consent, and most of the women who had the left hospital without knowing their pelvises had been broken. Many did not find out for decades. The side effects of symphysiotomy are horrific: incontinence, arthritis, and debilitating back pain, even the inability to walk.

Episiotomy was once routinely performed during every birth in the US. The risks, benefits, and alternatives for episiotomy have been heavily debated. Ideally, an episiotomy should be easily repairable incision when compared to uncontrolled vaginal trauma. It is still routinely performed in some countries.[90] The In 2005, a systematic review[91] in the *Journal of the American Medical Association* found no benefit to routine episiotomy[92] use. A 2017 Cochrane[93] review "could not identify any benefits of routine episiotomy for the baby or the mother." Today, the American College of Obstetricians and Gynecologists recommends that clinicians "prevent and manage" delivery lacerations through strategies like massage and warm compresses rather than making cuts on the perineum.

The first qualitative study[94] to examine mistreatment during childbirth in the US found that one in six women experience verbal abuse, stigma, discrimination, and being ignored when asking for help. The rates were even higher for non-white, younger, and/or lower income mothers. The

---

[90] Melo I, Katz L, Coutinho I, Amorim MM. "Selective episiotomy vs. implementation of a non-episiotomy protocol: a randomized clinical trial." *Reprod Health*. 2014 Aug 14;11:66.

[91] Hartmann K, Viswanathan M, Palmieri R, Gartlehner G, Thorp J, Lohr KN. "Outcomes of Routine Episiotomy: A Systematic Review." *JAMA*. 2005;293(17):2141–2148. doi:10.1001/jama.293.17.2141 https://jamanetwork.com/journals/jama/fullarticle/200799

[92] a surgical cut made at the opening of the vagina during childbirth, to aid a difficult delivery and prevent rupture of tissues.

[93] Jiang H, Qian X, Carroli G, Garner P. "Selective versus routine use of episiotomy for vaginal birth." Cochrane Database of Systematic Reviews 2017, Issue 2. Art. No.: CD000081. DOI: 10.1002/14651858.CD000081.pub3 https://www.cochrane.org/CD000081/PREG_selective-versus-routine-use-episiotomy-vaginal-birth.

[94] Vedam, S., Stoll, K., Taiwo, T.K. et al. "The Giving Voice to Mothers study: inequity and mistreatment during pregnancy and childbirth in the United States." *Reprod Health* 16, 77 (2019). https://doi.org/10.1186/s12978-019-0729-2. https://reproductive-health-journal.biomedcentral.com/articles/10.1186/s12978-019-0729-2.

most common type of mistreatment women reported in the survey was being shouted at or scolded by their doctors, midwives, or nurses. The next most common was being ignored by their health care providers, or having their requests refused or not responded to for a reasonable amount of time.

Disregard of consent during childbirth and the use of unwarranted interventions are more common than one might think. Mothers report experiencing pressure (feeling like they had "no choice") for a range of obstetric interventions, including; labor induction, epidurals, and C-sections.

Brazil has one of the highest Cesarean birth rates in the world.[95] The World Health Organization recommends a C-section rate of no more than 15%. In private Brazilian hospitals, the percentage hovers between 80 and 90%. Nationwide, the C-section rate is upward of 50%. By contrast, about 30% of American women undergo Cesarean births, and that rate is widely considered to be too high.

In Brazil, Cesarean sections are seen as "modern and elegant" for wealthy women who can afford to give birth in private facilities and have become a status symbol. If a woman wants a natural birth, it is almost viewed as an inconvenience for doctors, and they may find themselves going from hospital to hospital looking for a bed to give birth in because all the beds are full with scheduled births. Low-income women largely depend on the public health system, leading to much higher vaginal birth rates—which are viewed as primitive, ugly, nasty, inconvenient. As a result, most Brazilian women get C-sections, and Brazilian women feel pressured to acquiesce to this procedure, rather than personally choosing it.[96]

---

[95] Rudey, Edson Luciano et al. "Cesarean section rates in Brazil: Trend analysis using the Robson classification system." Medicine vol. 99,17 (2020): e19880. doi:10.1097/MD.0000000000019880 https://www.ncbi.nlm.nih.gov/pmc/articles/PMC7220553/.

[96] Potter, J, et al. "Unwanted caesarean sections among public and private patients in Brazil: prospective study" BMJ 2001; 323:1155. November 2011. https://www.bmj.com/content/323/7322/1155.

THE HUSBAND STITCH

The "husband stitch" (daddy stitch, husband's knot, or vaginal tuck) is a surgical procedure in which one or more sutures than necessary are used to repair a woman's perineum after it has been torn or cut during childbirth. The claimed purpose is to tighten the opening of the vagina and thereby enhance the pleasure of her male sex partner during penetrative intercourse, however there is no credible clinical evidence to support this practice. The husband stitch has been referred to in medical literature as far back as 1885, in Transactions of the Texas State Medical Association.[97] However, women who have their vaginal opening stitched too tightly can experience pain and dysfunction as a result. Ultimately, it seems as though some women themselves ask for an extra stitch, a good many more (anecdotally) feel they were given one without consent. An "extra stitch" given at the husband's request or because a physician thinks it will be helpful goes against surgical principles of healing.

The American Congress of Obstetricians and Gynecologists does not deny that the "husband stitch" procedure happens. However, its representatives claim that the practice "is not standard or common." There are no scientific studies that show how many women have been affected, nor is there a clear method for evaluating how prevalent the husband stitch truly is in obstetrics.

SHACKLED AND SEPARATED: PARTURITION IN PRISON

The shackling of pregnant prisoners during labor and childbirth is rampant within women's federal penal institutions in the United States, despite laws enacted in 21 states against the practice. Additionally, 46 states have no legislation that restrict the shackling of pregnant women in

---

[97] Transactions of the Texas State Medical Association. Seventeenth Annual Session. Houston, Texas: Texas State Medical Association. 21–23 April 1885.

jails, and detention centers, leaving the practice to the "discretion of individual facilities."

The United States has the highest incarceration rate of women in the world, with over 205,000 women currently committed to either state and federal prisons or jails, and another million on probation or parole.[98] The majority of women in prison and jail are in their reproductive years, with a median age of 34; it has been estimated that between 5-10% of women enter prison and jail pregnant, and approximately 2,000 babies are born to incarcerated women annually.[99]

When shackled, incarcerated women in labor experience the physical pain of giving birth while unable to move, the medical complications resulting from this lack of mobility (heightened risk of blood clots, increased the risk of falling, which can cause serious injury and even death), and the psychological distress of holding their newborns while chained to the hospital bed. In one recent case, a pretrial detainee named Tammy Jackson was ignored for hours while she went into active labor in her jail cell and was forced to suffer through the physical and emotional trauma of labor and delivery alone.

In addition to shackling, many pregnant women who deliver while incarcerated are almost immediately separated from their newborns after delivery. After giving birth, most incarcerated mothers are allowed only 24 hours with their newborns in the hospital; the infants are then either placed with relatives or in foster care, and the mothers are returned to prison or jail.

In one case, the ACLU of Nevada brought a case on behalf of a low-risk women incarcerated for a minor crime—stealing $250 worth of chips from a casino—who suffered pulled groin muscles and separated pubic bones from being shackled during labor, and within ten minutes of

---

[98] The Sentencing Project. Incarcerated women and girls. Updated November 2020. http://www.sentencingproject.org/doc/publications/cc_Incarcerated_Women_Factsheet_Dec2012final.pdf.

[99] Clarke, Jennifer G, and Eli Y Adashi. "Perinatal care for incarcerated patients: a 25-year-old woman pregnant in jail." *JAMA* vol. 305,9 (2011): 923-9. doi:10.1001/jama.2011.125. https://pubmed.ncbi.nlm.nih.gov/21304069/.

delivering via emergency C-section was placed back in ankle shackles and chained to the bed.

In another example of obstetric trauma, on July 31, 2018, an incarcerated woman was forced to give birth alone, with no medical supervision or treatment. Diana Sanchez was ignored for hours after she felt contractions about 5 a.m. on July 31, until after she gave birth at 10:44 a.m. At 10:45 a.m. a nurse called an ambulance, but the report indicates nurses didn't seem to know where to find a large clamp for the umbilical cord and had to call the Denver Fire Department to assist because paramedics were taking too long to arrive.

MIDWIVES

Midwifery care involves a trusting relationship between the provider and pregnant person, who share decision-making. Midwives also see pregnancy and labor as normal life processes rather than a condition to be managed.

Increasingly, US women are choosing to give birth outside of a hospital, at a birth center or at home and attended by a midwife. Substantial out-of-pocket costs associated with hospital births, the perception that homebirths are safer, with lower Cesarean rates and fewer interventions; increased patient empowerment and control of their own experience are driving the trend.

The rate of out-of-hospital births in the US has grown—29 percent between 2004 and 2009—according to the Centers for Disease Control and Prevention. There are different types of midwives, ranging from certified nurses with advanced degrees who deliver at hospitals to lay midwives, some of whom have no formal training but years of experience. Certified nurse-midwives (CNMs), who complete an extensive nursing education culminating in a graduate degree, can practice legally in all 50 states. But 28 states also allow "direct-entry" midwives, who may enter the profession through an apprenticeship to a more experienced midwife. As a result, the term "midwife" has no standardized meaning in the US.

Midwife-led maternity care is the norm in other developed countries, including most of Europe. Some areas of the US already lack enough obstetricians to meet demand, and the US will be short an estimated 9,000 obstetricians by 2030. The number of out-of-hospital births has increased from 35,578 in 2004 to 62,228 in 2017. In 2017, 1 of every 62 births in the US was an out-of-hospital birth (1.61%). Home births increased by 77% from 2004–2017, while birth center births have more than doubled.[100]

The rise of the natural birth industry, however, has led to what some believe is a failure to deliver good outcomes for women and babies. This is being investigated by journalists at Gatehouse Media. Their analysis shows that infants are three times more likely to die with midwife-assisted home births[101] than midwife-assisted hospital births. The risk climbs for babies of first-time mothers, who are four times more likely to die. When restricting the analysis to one week of age, the risk for first-born babies climbs eightfold.

However, we know that other developed countries see increased positive outcomes using the midwife model of care. Mothers whose care was led by a nurse-midwife were found to have lower rates of episiotomies, drug-induced labor, and vaginal tearing during delivery. Similarly, a 2013 Cochrane[102] review looked at hospital births in countries with advanced healthcare systems, including England, Australia, and Canada, and found that women whose care was led by a midwife rather than a physician were less likely to receive pain medication in labor, less likely to experience pre-term birth, and less likely to experience a miscarriage before 24 weeks gestation.

---

[100] MacDorman, Marian F, and Eugene Declercq. "Trends and state variations in out-of-hospital births in the United States, 2004-2017." *Birth* (Berkeley, Calif.) vol. 46,2 (2019): 279-288. doi:10.1111/birt.12411. https://www.ncbi.nlm.nih.gov/pmc/articles/PMC6642827/.
[101] https://github.com/GateHouseMedia/PLBID.
[102] Sandall J, Soltani H, Gates S, Shennan A, Devane D. Midwife-led continuity models versus other models of care for childbearing women. Cochrane Database of Systematic Reviews 2013, Issue 8. Art. No.: CD004667. DOI: 10.1002/14651858.CD004667.pub3. Accessed 29 November 2020. https://www.cochranelibrary.com/cdsr/doi/10.1002/14651858.CD004667.pub3/full.

The disparity in results in the US perhaps reflects the tension between obstetrics and midwifery and the wide ranges of pregnancy itself: it is *both* a normal natural process and a dangerous condition requiring care from highly trained specialists.

PREGNANCY CRISIS CENTERS

In the US, it is legal for fake doctors, posing in white lab coats, to lure desperate pregnant women into a fake reproductive health clinic for the sole purpose of misleading them about their health care options.

There is an entire pseudo healthcare industry that is dedicated to unethical and underhanded practices, which actively harm the health of women through deliberate and purposeful acts of misinformation.

Fake health centers, also known as crisis pregnancy centers, are unlicensed and unregulated facilities trying to prevent abortion through any means necessary. They aggressively mimic real OB/GYN offices: everything from their website to their branding to their interiors is indistinguishable from real clinics.

Fake reproductive health centers outnumber real women's health clinics by nearly 5:1. In the United States, there are about four fake health centers for every real abortion clinic; in Missouri, there is only one abortion provider and twenty-four fake clinics. That is because in a case known as *NIFLA v. Becerra* the five conservative justices of the Supreme Court ruled that anti-abortion "crisis pregnancy centers" should have heightened free speech protections that real doctors and abortion clinics do not.

The Supreme Court's majority opinion was articulated by Justice Clarence Thomas and outlined the Court's opinion that "Crisis Pregnancy Center" medical counselors do not actually provide medical counsel. Informed consent laws, the argument goes, apply *only to places that provide actual medical services*, not to fake pregnancy clinics that merely pretend to.

Thomas also noted that the same First Amendment protections do not apply to doctors in states like Mississippi and Arizona[103] who are required by the state to tell women false information about abortion, such as the supposed link between abortion and breast cancer, or that abortion is "reversible."

The National Cancer Institute, the American College of Obstetricians and Gynecologists, and the Collaborative Group on Hormonal Factors in Breast Cancer based out of Oxford University in England have found no evidence of a link between breast cancer and abortion, based on high-quality studies. Certainly, modern demographics, like birth control use, delayed childbirth, and obesity, combined with increased detection by mammography, overwhelmingly account for the rise in breast cancer diagnoses.[104]

Justice Stephen Breyer pointed out the hypocrisy in his dissent: "If a state can lawfully require a doctor to tell a woman seeking an abortion about adoption services," he wrote, "why should it not be able, as here, to require a medical counselor to tell a woman seeking prenatal care or other reproductive health care about childbirth and abortion services?"

Twenty-eight states require abortion clinics to carry state-written brochures containing information about alternatives to abortion, like adoption, and the supposed risks associated with the procedure, even if that information is not supported by science or medical research. Six states force doctors to inform women that abortion has serious mental health consequences, though studies by the American Psychological Association have shown that having an abortion has no more of an effect on mental health than continuing an unintended pregnancy to term. A handful of states force doctors to tell women that abortion jeopardizes future fertility, a claim without any science-based evidence, or that abortion can be reversed.

---

[103] "An Overview of Abortion Laws," Guttmacher Institute. https://www.guttmacher.org/state-policy/explore/overview-abortion-laws.

[104] Melbye, Mads, et al. "Induced Abortion and the Risk of Breast Cancer." *The New England Journal of Medicine*, January 1997. https://www.nejm.org/doi/pdf/10.1056/NEJM199701093360201.

Abortion reversal is not supported by medical science.[105] Essentially, our government is forcing doctors to recommend an experimental (and unproven) therapy, without making it clear that it's experimental.

The groundbreaking "Turnaway" Study[106] reveals the devastating effect of reproductive health-care denial, showing that women who are denied wanted abortions are more likely to suffer serious medical complications, including eclampsia and death, and mental health issues (anxiety and loss of self-esteem), or to stay with abusive partners. Women denied a wanted abortion who have to carry an unwanted pregnancy to term have four times greater odds of living below the Federal Poverty Level (FPL).

RACIAL DISPARITIES IN THE USA

The United States began tracking infant mortality rate by race in 1850. In over a century since then that gap, instead of shrinking with modern healthcare and sanitation, has actually *grown*. In 2017, Black newborns had twice the rate of infant mortality compared to the white non-Hispanic population. Black newborn infants die three times as often when taken care of by a white doctor than by a Black doctor. Additionally, Black women are four to five times more likely to die from pregnancy complications than white women. Lastly, married Black women are nearly twice as likely to experience infertility as married white women, but they are treated half as often, and are less likely to achieve pregnancy after *in vitro* fertilization (IVF), while suffering more severe complications and side effects (like ovarian hyperstimulation syndrome).

In 1850, the reported Black infant-mortality rate was 340 per 1,000; the white rate was 217 per 1,000. Today, in US-born Black infants are now

---

[105] "Facts are Important: Medication Abortion "Reversal" Is Not Supported by Science. The American College of Obstetricians and Gynecologists. https://www.acog.org/advocacy/facts-are-important/medication-abortion-reversal-is-not-supported-by-science.

[106] "Turnaway Study," University of California San Francisco. https://www.ansirh.org/research/turnaway-study.

more than twice as likely to die as white infants. This difference transcends class. A Black woman with an advanced degree is more likely to lose her baby than a white woman with less than an eighth-grade education. In this article, we will shed some light on lesser-known issues that, to this day, may cause trust issues between the medical community and the Black community. There are many well-known examples of unimaginable trust or consent breaches, such as the Tuskegee experiments, the story of Henrietta Lacks and HeLa cells, and the *Buck vs. Bell* decision and sterilization laws that targeted the poor and minorities to name just a few. Those events have been well covered and are beyond the scope of this article to discuss in a way that gives due justice to them.

These disparities (Black infant and maternal mortality, and lack of sexual health and fertility treatments) can start to be unraveled through an historical perspective of the history of gynecological and obstetrical violence and through examination of modern-day implicit biases that are deeply-rooted in society as a result of systemic racism.

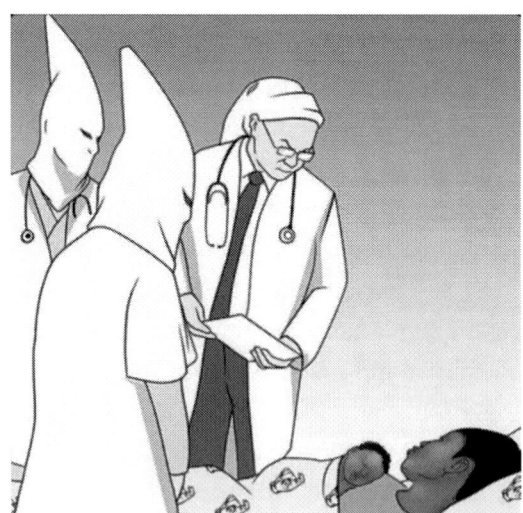

Image Source: Unknown.

Figure 10. Black newborn infants die three times as often when taken care of by a white doctor than by a Black doctor.

Black women are four to five times more likely to suffer pregnancy related mortality than white women. This statistic is only partially generated from Black women having a higher risk of pregnancy complications. The Centers for Disease Control and Prevention (CDC) stated that from 2007–2016, cardiomyopathy, thrombotic pulmonary embolism, and hypertensive disorders of pregnancy contributed more towards pregnancy-related mortalities in Black women than in white women. However, carefully conducted studies have shown that Black infant and maternal mortality cannot be fully explained by pre-existing medical conditions, *or* by income, weight, maternal vitamins, smoking, drinking, or drug use, or anything else—except for stress. The chronic, long term, toxic, unmanageable stress of being Black in America, the very inescapable atmosphere of societal and systemic racism that is cultivated here, leads directly to higher rates of infant and maternal death.

Lastly, we come to the undertreatment of infertility in Black women. One might assume that fewer Black women receiving treatment for infertility implies there are simply fewer Black women with infertility. It is definitely not that simple.

There are various explanations provided for the mistreatment of infertile people of color (POC). There are often misperceptions of POC being hyper-fertile or being unfit to be a mother. The trope of the "welfare queen" comes to mind as a strong visual, perpetrated by the media. A plump, lobster-eating, Cadillac driving, well dressed, Black or brown hyper-fertile woman, who has child after child to maintain the government handout.

Not only do historical racial inequities in medicine lead to inaccurate diagnoses, but there is also societal pressures and shame that result in a Black woman remaining silent about infertility struggles. It is not simply the societal views on infertility in Black women that are problematic, it's the greater need for investment in research and resources and the need to focus on racial disparity in assisted reproduction technology (ART) outcomes.

There is a marked, and unacceptable, difference in the outcomes after fertility treatment between populations:

- The ART failure rate (no live birth after treatment) is 51.9% (white), 61.8% (Asian), 62.2% (Black), and 55.9% (Hispanic).
- ART stillbirths are 16.3% (white), 18.4% (Asian), 25.0% (Black), and 17.8% (Hispanic).
- Tubal factor infertility diagnoses are 18.5% white women, 41.7% (non-Hispanic) Black women, 27.3% Hispanic women, and 17.0% Asian or Pacific Islander women.

The reasons these disparities exist includes genetics, income, health insurance, and maternal stress. However, there is a lack of outreach regarding accessible educational, counseling, and support resources to minority communities. Resources and education are what enable people to direct their sexual health and infertility care. Racial inequality and social stigma strip people of the power to do so. Historical stereotypes continue to stubbornly prevail and prohibit Black women from receiving the infertility healthcare and resources they require.

A study conducted by Ann V. Bell sheds some light on the subtle inequalities that play a role in treating infertility. Bell interviewed 27 women of low socioeconomic status. Ten participants were Black, two were Latina, and one was Asian. The findings of her research were disturbing and demonstrate how ethnic communities do not have pleasant, welcoming, and helpful doctor visits. For example, one 33-year-old Black woman interviewed by Bell recounted her experience after suffering a miscarriage:

> "They—they just—they just seem like they just didn't want me to have any kids (laughs) at all. At all. And that was sad. They, you know, they scared me into even trying to have any more. They tried—they tried to get me not to even have any more […] They was really scaring me. That's why I—I said, 'Oh (laughs). Never again, Holy Grace Hospital. Never again.' Because they scared me, and it was just—just crazy."

I interviewed the founder of the Fibroid Pandemic, LaToya Dwight, BBA, MSM, RHU, ChCC, REBC. The Fibroid Pandemic is a support group for women with fibroids (especially for POC, who get little support). When Ms. Dwight's white doctor diagnosed her fibroids, they immediately prescribed a hysterectomy (removal of the uterus). Obviously, that is a huge, life changing decision; yet, despite the gravity of it, the treatment plan was handed down cavalierly with no mutual discussion or consent, and no discussion of alternate, fertility preservation options. She changed physicians (to a Black doctor) and discovered that there are other, less severe options—diet and lifestyle changes and embolization, among others.

Not even fame and wealth can prevent Black women from experiencing these inequalities. Celebrities like Gabrielle Union and Serena Williams have publicly shared their infertility and post-birth near death experiences. Gabrielle Union struggled with heavy periods, pain, and infertility for years, before one doctor took her symptoms seriously and finally, accurately diagnosed her adenomyosis. Prior to that, every doctor simply dismissed her concerns and put her on birth control pills. After giving birth to her son, Serena Williams suffered a life-threatening blood clot in her lungs. Unfortunately, at first the medical staff did not believe her, but eventually a CT scan proved her right—she had a pulmonary embolism and several small blood clots had traveled to her lungs.

The above-mentioned inequalities are appalling alone, however, the picture gets bleaker still for Black newborns. Black newborns are more likely to survive in hospital if taken care by Black doctors. This was unequivocally demonstrated by an analysis of 1.8 million hospital births in Florida between 1992–2015.[107] In 2017, the CDC data also backs up the fact that Black newborns have twice the rate of infant mortality compared to white non-Hispanics. Neonatal mortality rate is the highest among Black non-Hispanic newborns.

---

[107] Brad N. Greenwood, Rachel R. Hardeman, Laura Huang, Aaron Sojourner. "Physician–patient racial concordance and disparities in birthing mortality for newborns."
Proceedings of the National Academy of Sciences, Sep 2020, 117 (35) 21194-21200; DOI: 10.1073/pnas.1913405117 https://www.pnas.org/content/117/35/21194.

Chapter 6

GENDER

THE ORIGIN OF FEMALE AND MALE REPRODUCTIVE TRACTS

Early philosophers often described the male and female reproductive tracts and organs like they were one entity with no distinct difference in features, such that the female reproductive tract was described using the male reproductive tract as a yardstick.

The philosopher Galen (200 AD), stated that all the parts that men possess, women possess too. He thought that the only difference between the male and the female reproductive tracts was that in men, these parts were outside in an area called the perineum, while for the women, their parts were located within the body. The use of male features to describe the female reproductive tract anatomy continued into the middle ages with other prominent early scientists like Master Nicolaus, ca. 1150-1200. He described the testes and ovary as if they were the same; in his words, the testes are moist in complexion and hot; the testes are further described as soft and delicate and spongy in composition. Master Nicolaus also described these reproductive organs "Testes" as large in men and small in the female. These "testes" produced sperm in both males and females.

As time passed, knowledge about the male and female reproductive anatomy increased. Several notable pre-vesalian anatomists produced more descriptive pictures of the reproductive tracts. Alessandro Achillini was able to depict the internal architecture of the female reproductive tract. Although he still called the ovaries testicles, he said the seminal vessels descend to the uterus and just outside it. These seminal vessels were interwoven near her "testicles," this network of interwoven mass was filled with glandular flesh.

Alessandro Benedetti (1497) further stressed the time's definition of a male and a female as relying solely on the possession of the testicles, such that when they are removed through castration, those individuals are not considered male anymore but female, because they lose their strength, beards, and "manly" habits.

Leonardo Da Vinci opined on the anatomical representation of the male reproductive tract. The starting point of the penis was to be positioned directly on the pubic bone. As a result, it can resist its active force during sexual intercourse. According to Da Vinci, in a situation where this bone is missing, during coitus, the penis, encountering resistance would consequently turn backward/inwards such that it would go into the body of the male, more than into that of the body of the individual at the other end. However, according to Da Vinci's account, the female reproductive tract has two "spermatic vessels" shaped like testicles, while her "sperm" initially was thought to be blood. But when insemination takes place, the female "testicles" welcome the generative faculty. By 1694, human sperm were observed through a microscope and the Spermist theory of reproduction claimed little fully formed men existed inside sperm.

Early scientists, despite the technological deficit in terms of advanced tools and instruments, were able to understand the reproductive traits. Still, they were limited in the description and terms used for these descriptions. Scholars at this time were able to paint a clear picture of reproduction, although the terms they chose to use limited these views into a "one-sex" model with the female not given full recognizance and "autonomy."

Gender 67

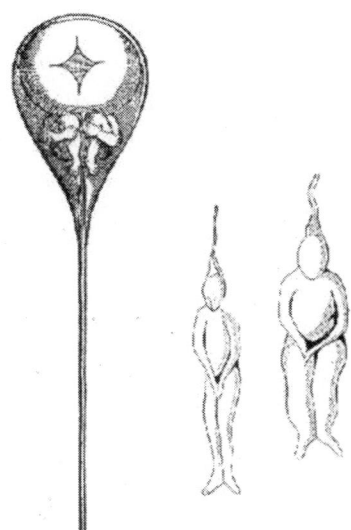

Image Source: Wikimedia Commons.
https://en.wikipedia.org/wiki/Nicolaas_Hartsoeker#/media/File:Preformation.GIF.

Figure 11. Illustration of homunculi in sperm, drawn by Nicolaas Hartsoeker in 1695.

DEVELOPMENT OF THE REPRODUCTIVE TRACTS

The development of the reproductive tract starts immediately after fertilization of the oocyte has taken place; the primordial gonads start development at about four weeks after conception. Reproductive tract development carries on in utero; however, little change occurs in the reproductive system between infancy and puberty. The reproductive tract comprises the structures resulting from the Müllerian ducts for females, while the ones derived from the Wolffian ducts are for males.

The development of the male and female reproductive systems is distinctively achieved by the fundamental molecular processes found across species. These processes at the primary stages are wholly unconnected with the sex of the growing offspring.

They give sexually neutral structures the capacity to develop into either male or female reproductive tracts. In other words, the male and female embryos both develop Wolffian ducts and Müllerian ducts, respectively, during their growth/development. Still, just one of these two will go on to survive and develop into a working reproductive tract.

Reproductive (Sex) Organs Development

Shortly after the conception of a zygote by fertilization, the reproductive tract development process starts and goes on all through gestation for viviparous (live-birth) animals and incubation for oviparous (egg-laying) animals. The timeline of these periods differs from species to species. In humans, it takes 2–8 weeks of the embryonic period for gestation to take place, while the remaining 32 weeks are termed the fetal period. Interestingly, the development is not complete until after birth, up to progression into adolescents who are finally mature into adults with the capability to sexually reproduce.

Females are deemed the "fundamental" sex because, with no copious chemical instigation, all oocytes fertilized would naturally develop as female. Also, the external genitalia in females autonomously develops in the fetus, thus requiring no hormonal instigation at this phase. The general genetic control of testis and ovarian differentiation hinges on SRY (Sex Related gene on the Y chromosome), which is the testes determining factor gene. The SRY is expressed in the intermediate mesoderm after embryonic development. In both female and male embryos, the same cluster of cells has the capacity to either develop into the male or female gonads; this is deemed "bi-potential." To become a male, the fertilized oocyte must be subjected to the gush of factors instigated by a particular single gene on the male Y chromosome—the SRY. Because females do not possess a Y chromosome, consequently they do not possess the SRY gene. And in the absence of a functional SRY gene, such a person will be female.

Male Reproductive Tract

As soon as the testes start differentiation after SRY, testosterone is secreted by the fetal Leydig cells, and Müllerian Inhibiting Substance (MIS) is released by Sertoli cells. These two hormones carry out broadly contrasting roles and processes; however, only the combination of their actions creates a normal male reproductive tract. Testosterone affixes to its intracellular receptor and acts as a transcriptional regulator that brings about the Wolffian duct's differentiation and proliferation to give the epididymis, seminal vesicles, and vas deferens. Without the testosterone or the absence of its functional receptor, this proliferation and differentiation do not occur. These receptors are initially present in the budding duct's mesenchyme. The processes and mechanisms of these cells, most probably by paracrine process in reaction to androgen, leads the epithelial cell compartment to its appropriate end.

Female Reproductive Tract

In the absence of testes and consequently MIS and testosterone, the Müllerian ducts develop into the uterus cervix, Fallopian tubes, and the upper part of the vagina. The coelomic epithelium invaginates to develop into the Müllerian duct and covers the ovaries. One of the final steps in fetal reproductive tract development for both sexes is the final positioning of the gonads. The ovaries remain in the pelvis while the testes descend into the scrotum.

There are rare and fascinating reproductive tract related developmental abnormalities.

About 1% to 5% of female infants are born with ectopic or "accessory" breast tissue. This rare condition is caused by remnants of the mammary ridges that fail to involute during embryologic development. To date, only less than 100 cases have been reported in the literature worldwide, and even rarer still 39 cases have been reported of ectopic breast tissue in the vulva. Ectopic breast tissue can respond to lactation hormones after pregnancy.

In Dominican Republic, Turkey, and New Guinea, some children literally appear to change their sex when they hit adolescence. Raised as girls, they grow a penis and testicles when they hit puberty, around the age of 12. When they're born, they look like girls with no testes and what appears to be a vagina; it is only when they near puberty that the penis grows, and testicles descend. A deficiency in the enzyme 5-α-reductase, means the body doesn't create the male sex hormone dihydrotestosterone (DHT), which prevents the development of male sex organs, until puberty hits, at least, when increased levels of testosterone belatedly reveal that Guevedoces (as they are called in Dominican Republic) are male.

Mayer-Rokitansky-Küster-Hauser (MRKH) syndrome is a rare disorder that affects women. It is characterized by the failure of the uterus and the vagina to develop properly in women who have normal ovarian function and normal external genitalia.

GENETICS, SEX, AND GENDER

The X and Y chromosomes are both originally derived from autosomes (all the other non sex related chromosomes) and were initially about the same size. Genetic deterioration of the Y chromosome has occurred because unlike with the two X chromosomes in women, there is very little swapping of genetic material between the Y and X chromosome during reproduction. This quickly led to a catastrophic deterioration of the Y chromosome, which now contains only 3 percent of the genes that it once shared with the X chromosome. This also means that mutations and deletions in the Y chromosome are preserved between (male) generations. The X chromosome bears more than 1,000 genes. But the Y has fewer than 80 functional genes. However, the Y chromosome is not all male-specific; 24 genes at the chromosome tips are still shared with the X chromosome, and those are the current sites of recombination during meiosis.

One of the genes that are not shared is the sex-determining region Y gene (SRY), which kick-starts the pathway that causes a ridge of cells in a 12-week-old embryo to develop into a testis.

Although the Y chromosome's role in sex determination is clear, research has shown that it is still undergoing rapid evolutionary deterioration. This has led to debates and concerns over the years regarding the Y chromosome's eventual destiny. Several groups have speculated that the Y chromosome has become superfluous and could completely decay within the next 10 million years. Animal don't need sex chromosomes after all. All of our other chromosomes are a mix of sex-related and non sex-related genes. It seems unlikely that the Y chromosome will disappear entirely. While the rate of deterioration was high 100 million or more years ago, the human Y chromosome has lost only one gene since humans and rhesus monkeys diverged evolutionarily 25 million years ago. It hasn't lost any genes since the divergence of chimpanzees 6 million years ago.[108]

Until recently, many believed that only the presence or absence of SRY is needed to distinguish males from females. However, we now know from case studies that there are significant gaps in our scientific knowledge of exactly how gender is specified in the developing embryo.

For example, genetically female (XX) *yet* SRY negative AND phenotypically male individuals prove that we don't know all the ways "sex" occurs. Out of all known cases of genotypically XX but phenotypically males, in up to 10 % of cases the SRY gene is not actually present. We do not know the exact cause of this condition, but it seems as if SOX9 gene (plays a role in the development of the testes) mutations contribute. Another proposed cause is mutations to the DAX1 (a nuclear hormone receptor) which represses masculinizing genes, therefore, if there is a loss of function of DAX1 then testes can develop in a genetically XX individual. Mutations in SF1 and WNT4 genes are also being studied in connection with SRY-negative XX male syndrome.

---

[108] Hughes, J., Skaletsky, H., Pyntikova, T. et al. Conservation of Y-linked genes during human evolution revealed by comparative sequencing in chimpanzee. Nature 437, 100–103 (2005). https://doi.org/10.1038/nature04101 https://www.nature.com/articles/nature04101.

Another variation is found in a case report of a genetically "male" XY individual, but who has "complete gonadal dysgenesis"—meaning that the woman underwent spontaneous puberty, reached menarche, menstruated regularly, and experienced two unassisted pregnancies. Additionally, she gave birth to a 46,XY daughter, also with complete gonadal dysgenesis.

"Herein we report the extraordinary case of a fertile woman with normal ovaries and a predominantly 46,XY ovarian karyotype, who gave birth to a 46,XY female with complete gonadal dysgenesis."[109]

Conventionally, because the gonads are dysgenetic they should also be nonfunctional, spontaneous pubertal development seldom occurs in these women, and successful pregnancy is even more unusual; unassisted pregnancy was unheard of until this case.

With the advent of affordable and easy DNA sequencing and the connectivity of the world through the internet, we now know there are dozens of variations in genetics that prove we have only the barest grasp of how sex is actually determined. Every 1 in 9000 to 1 in 20,000 human males has a 46,XX genotype. They are phenotypically sterile males with normal female chromosomes. We can now identify two forms of this syndrome: Y DNA positive and Y DNA negative. The Y DNA positive males result from a X;Y translocation with a low recurrence risk; the Y DNA negative males are due to a mutation with a high recurrence risk.[110]

Biological sex and gender are different; gender is not inherently nor solely connected to one's physical anatomy. Most people believe that our gender identity (the conviction of belonging to the male or female gender) and sexual orientation (who we are sexually attracted to) should be programmed into our brain structures when we are still in the womb.

During pregnancy, the fetal brain develops in the male direction through the direct action of testosterone on the developing nerve cells, or in the female direction through the absence of this hormone. Sexual differentiation of the genitals takes place in the first two months of

---

[109] Dumic, Miroslav et al. "Report of fertility in a woman with a predominantly 46,XY karyotype in a family with multiple disorders of sexual development." The Journal of clinical endocrinology and metabolism vol. 93,1 (2008): 182-9. doi:10.1210/jc.2007-2155 https://www.ncbi.nlm.nih.gov/pmc/articles/PMC2190741/.

[110] https://journals.sagepub.com/doi/abs/10.1177/000992289103000103.

pregnancy. Sexual differentiation of the brain, by contrast, starts in the second half of pregnancy. Therefore, these two processes are not linked to each other. They occur independently. Every animal starts off with two sets of organs, one that can become a male reproductive tract and one that can become a female reproductive tract. Every single person at one point in their life was a hermaphrodite.

The accepted medical treatment for an individual with gender dysphoria is not to attempt changing the brain, but to help the individual bring their physical body in line with the way they feel. There is no medically acceptable way to convince someone that they should feel a certain gender, even the gender they are genetically. Hence, gender reassignment surgeries or any other method people prefer to bring their body in line about their gender feeling.

There are many common genetic differences from the XY chromosome set, and many people do not even know that they have a genetic variance. For example:

- A genetically XY male's testicles may not descend. At birth it would be assumed in the absence of a genetic test, that this is a girl.
- XXY individuals are infertile males who have two X chromosomes.
- XY males can be born with a mutation in the cell receptor, i.e., the lock for the key testosterone. This disorder can be full or partial, and it is called androgen insensitivity syndrome.

Additionally, "male" and "female" hormones are unfortunately named because testosterone and estrogen are made from the same molecule, cholesterol. The progenitor molecule is whittled down and added to, each step removes or adds a piece; cortisol the "stress" hormone comes first, then testosterone is made, then estrogen. All from the same molecules, which are present in both males and females.

OFFICIAL DOCUMENTS

Lucy Hicks Anderson (1886–1954) was assigned male at birth but was adamant that she was a girl from an early age. Luckily for Lucy, her parents and doctors fully supported her gender transition by the time she started school. She got married and became a renowned chef, preparing dinner parties for the area's elite. After divorcing her husband, she made a living operating a brothel where she also sold liquor during prohibition. She was able to get away with these illegal activities thanks to her reputation as a socialite. In fact, the one time she was arrested for selling liquor, a friend bailed her out because he needed her help with a dinner party, he was hosting that very evening. In 1944, she married her second husband, a soldier named Reuben Anderson. The next year, trouble began when a sailor visited her brothel and contracted an STI, leading to an outbreak in the US Navy.

Lucy and all the women working in the brothel were legally required to undergo a medical examination. The exam revealed that Lucy was a transgender woman, and since this was an era where trans people could not have their gender legally recognized, she was charged with perjury for registering as female on her marriage license and put on trial. Her most famous quote comes from that trial: "I defy any doctor in the world to prove that I am not a woman." She was found guilty and sentenced to ten years' probation.

The federal government was not satisfied with probation and, because they no longer recognized the validity of the Andersons' marriage, sent both Lucy and Reuben to prison for Lucy having "fraudulently" collected money allotted to soldiers' wives. While in prison, Lucy was forced to wear male clothes. After their release, the couple moved to Los Angeles where they lived happily until Lucy's death. Today, Lucy is regarded as one of the earliest known African American transgender people.

There's a difference between sex and gender, but we conflate those on official documents. If all citizens are treated equally under the law anyway, then why does the government need to know your gender? Of course, laws and policies do use gender to discriminate on the basis of sex. The United States Supreme Court did not even recognize that the constitution prohibits discrimination based on gender until 1971.

At least 10 countries—Australia, Bangladesh, Canada, Denmark, Germany, India, Malta, Nepal, New Zealand and Pakistan—offer gender-neutral options on passports or national identity cards.

The governments of both India (1994)[111] and Pakistan (2009)[112] have recognized hijras as a "third sex," thus granting them the basic civil rights of every citizen. In India, hijras now have the option to identify as a eunuch ("E") on passports and on certain government documents. They are not, however, fully accommodated; in order to vote, for example, citizens must identify as either male or female. Other countries have no mechanism to recognize any option other than male or female. In order to obtain a birth certificate in Kenya, for example, a sex needs to be assigned to a child. Without that, children cannot enroll in school, or obtain a passport or identity document.

In an extreme example, Japan's Supreme Court recently upheld a law[113] that effectively requires transgender people to be sterilized before they can have their gender changed on official documents. The 2004 law states that people wishing to register a gender change must have their original reproductive organs, including testes or ovaries, removed and have a body that "appears to have parts that resemble the genital organs" of the gender they want to register. The court said the law is constitutional because it was meant to reduce confusion in families and society. It acknowledged that it restricts freedom and could become out of step with changing social values.

---

[111] "Politicians of the third gender: the "shemale" candidates of Pakistan." *New Statesman.*
[112] Usmani, Basim (18 July 2009). "Pakistan to register 'third sex' hijras." *The Guardian.*
[113] https://www.nbcnews.com/feature/nbc-out/japan-s-supreme-court-upholds-transgender-sterilization-requirement-n962721.

INTERSEX TIMELINE

- 2013 The UN special rapporteur on torture says non-consensual "genital normalising surgery arguably meets the criteria for torture"
- 2015 Malta becomes the first country to ban non-consensual modifications to sex characteristics
- 2017 Human Rights Watch and interACT call for a moratorium on all safely deferrable surgical procedures on children with atypical sex characteristics
- 2018 Germany adopts intersex identity into law, people can register as intersex on birth certificates and passports from 1 January 2019
- 2019 a UK task force of NHS doctors and intersex activists is assembled to look into informed consent and surgery on children

CONVERSION THERAPY

Countries around the world use a range of so called "corrective" coercive therapies targeted at changing the sexuality of individuals, these include (but are not limited to); psychological coercion, solitary confinement, prayer, starvation, beatings, and torture. Outright International's report[114] shows how "conversion therapy" is a worldwide phenomenon. The report draws on data from an extensive literature review, the first-ever global survey on the topic, and in-depth interviews with experts and survivors from various countries. The premise of conversion therapy is that same sex attraction and the spectrum of gender identity are considered disordered and therefore in need of "cure," "repair," or counseling to regain a heterosexual or cisgender identity. The report represents the first time that the nature and extent of these damaging,

---

[114] https://outrightinternational.org/reports/global-reach-so-called-conversion-therapy

degrading practices globally has been documented. The report traces an organized and internationally connected ultra-conservative and religious right movement and global backlash to the rights that have been gained in the last 30 years. There is clear evidence that conversion therapy does not work, and significant evidence that it is harmful to lesbian, gay, bi, trans, and queer (LGBTQ) people.[115]

Conversion therapy is banned nationwide in Brazil, Ecuador, and Malta. While it is illegal in Ecuador, gay people, particularly lesbians, are forced to undergo conversion therapy in secret clinics.

Although there is no federal ban in Canada, nearly half the population lives in regions with local laws prohibiting the practice.

Brutal and extreme conversion methods including torture, forced internment, electroshock therapy and sexual violence have been documented in Ecuador, South Africa, the Dominican Republic, and China.

Laws in Argentina, Fiji, and Samoa do not specifically ban conversion therapy but prohibit any medical diagnosis based exclusively on a person's sexual orientation.

Britain's state-run National Health Service has signed a memorandum of understanding that opposes conversion therapy.

United States

To date, California, Colorado, Connecticut, Delaware, Hawaii, Illinois, Maine, Maryland, Massachusetts, Nevada, New Hampshire, New Jersey, New Mexico, New York, Oregon, Rhode Island, Utah, Virginia, Vermont, Washington, the District of Columbia, and Puerto Rico all have laws or regulations protecting youth from this harmful practice.

A growing number of municipalities have also enacted similar protections, including at least 70 cities and counties in Arizona, Colorado,

---

[115] "Resolution on Appropriate Affirmative Responses to Sexual Orientation Distress and Change Efforts. American Psychological Association. 2009. https://www.apa.org/about/policy/sexual-orientation.

Florida, Georgia, Iowa, Kentucky, Michigan, Minnesota, Missouri, New York, Ohio, Pennsylvania, Washington, and Wisconsin.

The Gender Expression Non-Discrimination Act (GENDA) is a 2019 New York law which added gender identity and gender expression to the state's human rights and hate crimes laws as protected classes; banned discrimination in employment, housing, and public accommodations based on gender identity and gender expression; and provided enhanced penalties for bias-motivated crimes. GENDA was first introduced in 2003.[116] The bill passed the New York State Assembly every year from 2008 to 2019 but was not passed by each house of the New York State Legislature until January 15, 2019.

New York Gov. Andrew Cuomo signed it into law on January 25, 2019 saying, "By signing into law GENDA and a ban on the fraudulent practice of conversion therapy, we are taking another giant step forward in advancing equal justice for every New Yorker, regardless of their gender identity or sexual orientation. We are once again sending a clear and proud message that there is no place for hate in our state, and anyone who engages in bigotry and discrimination will be held accountable."

On three separate occasions—April 2019, February 2016, and May 2015—the Supreme Court of the United States (SCOTUS) upheld New Jersey's anti-conversion therapy law to remain in effect. They also refused to hear challenges to California's anti-conversion therapy law essentially, affirming the law's constitutionality.

SEX SELECTION

Sex selection is the attempt to control the sex of the offspring to achieve a desired sex. It can be accomplished in several ways, both pre- and post-implantation of an embryo, as well as horrifically, at childbirth.

---

[116] Robert Harding. "NY Legislature OKs transgender rights bill, GENDA, after years-long effort." Auburn Citizen.

The application of these techniques to humans creates moral and ethical concerns in the opinion of some, while the advantages of sensible use of selected technologies is favored by others.

Sex-selection technology providers (those who perform *in vitro* fertilization and preimplantation genetic testing) generally argue that sex selection is an expression of reproductive rights, it is initiated and pursued by women, and is a sign of female empowerment that allows couples to make well-informed family planning decisions, it prevents the occurrences of unintended pregnancy and abortion, and minimizes intimate partner violence and/or child neglect.

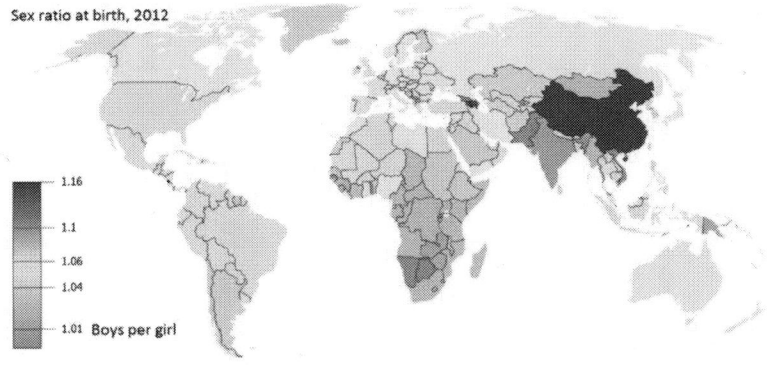

Image Source: Wikimedia Commons.
https://en.wikipedia.org/wiki/Sex_selection#/media/File:2012_Birth_Sex_Ratio_World_Map.jpg.

Figure 12. World map of birth sex ratios, 2012.

Severe sex-ratio imbalances as a result of new sex-selection technologies (ultrasound, preimplantation genetic diagnostics) are currently affecting many countries worldwide, including India, China, South Korea, among others.[117] Cultural son-preference combined with

---

[117] Hesketh, Therese et al. "The consequences of son preference and sex-selective abortion in China and other Asian countries." CMAJ : Canadian Medical Association journal = journal de l'Association medicale canadienne vol. 183,12 (2011): 1374-7. doi:10.1503/cmaj.101368 https://www.ncbi.nlm.nih.gov/pmc/articles/PMC3168620/.

forced small family size policies, have led to infanticide, forced abortion, under registration of female births, and death due to neglect and starvation.

In China, son preference and sex-selective abortion have led to 32 million excess males under the age of 20 years.

Men for whom marriage is unavailable are assumed to be psychologically vulnerable (not being able to participate in society, low self-esteem from not marrying and having a family, sexual frustration) and may be prone to aggression and violence.

Policy makers are addressing some causes of the high sex ratio at birth, but more could be done.

Governments realize that nothing can realistically be done to reduce the current excess of young males, but much has to be done to reduce sex selection now.

Chapter 7

GENITAL ALTERATION

GENITAL CUTTING

Children, whether male, female, or intersex, should be protected from having parts of their genitals removed, modified, nicked, scraped, or modified for any purpose other than a pressing medical indication. Female Genital Mutilation (FGM) and male circumcision are practiced throughout nearly every culture, by many religious faiths (Jewish, Christian, Muslim, and many more), at many stages of development from infancy through puberty, range from (mostly) benign and symbolic to extremely harmful (life-long health problems, mutilation, infection, and death), and are performed by a range of individuals from skilled medical professionals in sterile clinical settings to lay-practitioners using unsterile objects like thorns or glass shards. Throughout history until now, these procedures have been performed for a wide variety of reasons: to mark the initiation into a religious tradition, to mark the transition between childhood and adulthood around the time of puberty, to treat hypersexuality (insanity, sexual urges and pleasure, masturbation), and a current worrisome trend in Western countries, for cosmetic reasons, as teenage girls can undergo labiaplasty and vaginal tucks.

The World Health Organization condemns all forms of female genital cutting—no matter how minor—as mutilations, and all Western democracies prohibit them; however, male genital cutting is not prohibited anywhere, and in many places no restrictions or rules govern it. Anyone with any amount of training (including none), using any instrument (from sterile to mouth/teeth), can perform circumcisions on unanesthetized and unconsenting children.

We tend to think of female genital cutting as a horrific and aberrant practice and only as the harshest type, performed in the dirtiest, worst conditions, and leading to the worst outcomes. We tend to think of male genital cutting as hygienic, safe, and perhaps even morally and philosophically permissible to make a male child resemble their father. These are biased errors in thinking. Certainly, in some cultures what happens to boys is worse[118] than what happens to girls, and vice versa. For example, at puberty, the penis may be incised, and the urethra slit open lengthwise. In many cultures, boys are circumcised while fully conscious and with the expectation that they will not utter a sound, where bearing the pain is a critical test of masculinity.[119] Even among clinical settings the risks of severe to fatal hemorrhaging, infection, and mutilation of the penis exist.[120]

Around the 19th and 20th centuries female genital cutting was regularly performed in the US and England[121] as a legitimate medical procedure, to treat health issues, masturbation in young girls, and to help husbands find the clitoris of adult married women. Sometimes, clitorectomies were performed at the requests of the women's husbands or

---

[118] Peltzer, K., Nqeketo, A., Petros, G. et al. "Traditional circumcision during manhood initiation rituals in the Eastern Cape, South Africa: a pre-post intervention evaluation." *BMC Public Health* 8, 64 (2008). https://bmcpublichealth.biomedcentral.com/articles/10.1186/1471-2458-8-64.

[119] "32 boys dead in S.African initiation season," Medical Express. https://medicalxpress.com/news/2015-07-boys-dead-safrican-season.html

[120] El Bcheraoui C, Zhang X, Cooper CS, Rose CE, Kilmarx PH, Chen RT. "Rates of Adverse Events Associated With Male Circumcision in US Medical Settings, 2001 to 2010." *JAMA Pediatr.* 2014;168(7):625–634. doi:10.1001/jamapediatrics.2013.5414. https://jamanetwork.com/journals/jamapediatrics/fullarticle/1870232

[121] Sarah W. Rodriguez. "Rethinking the History of Female Circumcision and Clitoridectomy: American Medicine and Female Sexuality in the Late Nineteenth Century." *Journal of the History of Medicine and Allied Sciences*, Volume 63, Issue 3, July 2008, Pages 323–347. https://doi.org/10.1093/jhmas/jrm044 https://academic.oup.com/jhmas/article-abstract/63/3/323/816601.

fathers, who were permitted under the law to commit the women to surgery involuntarily. In fundamentalist Christian communities there is evidence that that female genital cutting is still performed today.[122]

A common universal impact of female genital cutting is difficulty giving birth and relates to the extent of the genital cutting, because genital scar tissue does not stretch, it can cause obstruction and tearing of the tissues around the vagina during childbirth, which prolongs labor and increases the risk of caesarean section. Women with scar tissue are also more likely to undergo episiotomy, heavy bleeding, and distress in the newborn infant and stillbirth.[123]

SEX REASSIGNMENT SURGERY

One of the first recorded examples in the US of gender-norm violation, involved a servant in the Virginia colony in the 1620s, who claimed to be both a man and a woman and at different times adopted the traditional roles and clothing of both men and women. This individual went by the names of Thomas and Thomasine Hall. Unable to establish Hall's "true" gender, despite repeated physical examinations, and unsure of whether to punish him/her for wearing men's or women's apparel, local citizens asked the court at Jamestown to resolve the issue.

Perhaps because it too was unable to make a conclusive determination, or maybe because it took Hall at his/her word that Hall was bi-gendered or what would be known today as intersex, the court ordered Hall in 1629 to wear both a man's breeches and a woman's apron and cap. This unique ruling affirmed Hall's dual nature. It subverted traditional gender categories, but by fixing Hall's gender and denying him/her the freedom to switch between male and female identities, the decision simultaneously

---

[122] Bergstrom, A Renee, "FGM happened to me in white, midwest America," The Guardian, December 2016. https://www.theguardian.com/us-news/2016/dec/02/fgm-happened-to-me-in-white-midwest-america

[123] "New study shows female genital mutilation exposes women and babies to significant risk at childbirth," World Health Organization. https://www.who.int/mediacentre/news/releases/2006/pr30/en/.

punished Hall and reinforced gender boundaries. It also forever marked Hall publicly as an oddity in the Virginia settlement, and likely made him/her the subject of ridicule and pity.[124] Reflecting how dominant gender expectations had changed little in the intervening three hundred years, another individual named Hall would confound authorities at the turn of the twentieth century. Murray Hall lived as a man for thirty years, becoming a prominent New York City politician, operating a commercial "intelligence office," and marrying twice. Hall was not discovered to have been assigned Female at birth until his death in 1901 from breast cancer, for which he had avoided medical treatment for several years, seemingly out of a fear that the gender assigned to him at birth would become public. His wives were aware of Hall's secret and respected how he expressed his gender. No one else knew, including the daughter he raised, and his friends and colleagues were shocked at the revelation.

While some officials and a coroner's jury subsequently chose to see Hall as Female, his daughter, friends, and political colleagues continued to recognize him as a man. Said an aide to a New York State Senator, "If he was a woman he ought to have been born a man, for he lived and looked like one."[125] Hirschfeld's Institute for Sexual Science, the world's first institute devoted to sexology, also performed the earliest recorded genital transformation surgeries. The first documented case was that of Dorchen Richter, a male-assigned individual from a poor German family who had desired to be female since early childhood, lived as a woman when she could, and hated her male anatomy. She underwent castration in 1922 and had her penis removed and a vagina constructed in 1931.

Following her first surgery, Richter was given a job at the institute as a domestic worker and served as an example for other patients.[126] The institute's most well-known patient was Einar Wegener, a Dutch painter who began to present and identify as Lili Elbe in the 1920s, and after being

---

[124] Brown, K. (1995). "Changed . . . into the fashion of man": The politics of sexual difference in a seventeenth-century Anglo-American settlement. *Journal of the History of Sexuality*, 6 (21), 171-93.
[125] Cromwell, J. (1999). Transmen and FTMs: Identities, bodies, genders, and sexualities. Urbana: University of Illinois Press.
[126] Hoyer, Niels, *Man Into Woman*, Popular Library, New York, 1953.

evaluated by Hirschfeld, underwent a series of male-to-female surgeries. In addition to castration and the construction of a vagina, she had ovaries inserted into her abdomen, which at a time before the synthesis of hormones, was the only way that doctors knew to try to change estrogen levels. It is extremely doubtful that the operation had any real effect. Still, Elbe felt that it made her both a woman and young again and proceeded with a final surgery to create a uterus in an attempt to be a mother and no different from other women.[127] She died from heart failure in 1931 in the aftermath of the surgery.

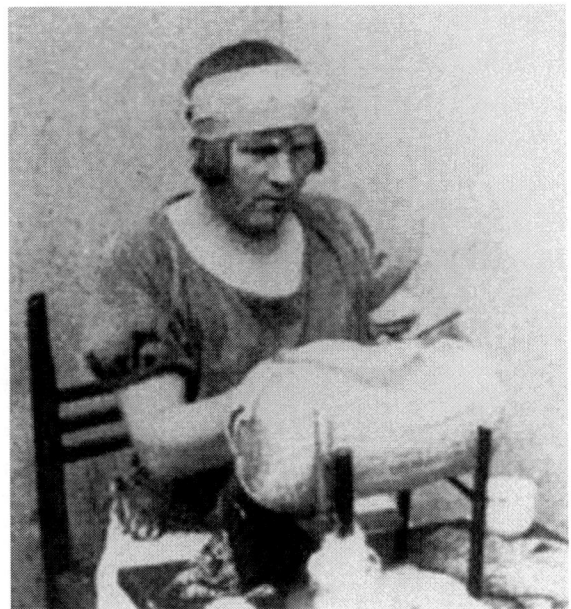

Image Source: Wikimedia Commons.
https://en.wikipedia.org/wiki/Dora_Richter#/media/File:DoraRichter.png.

Figure 13. Dörchen Richter, was the first known person to undergo complete male-to-female gender reassignment surgery.

---

[127] Hoyer, Niels, *Man Into Woman*, Popular Library, New York, 1953.

Before her death, though, Elbe requested that her friend Ernst Ludwig Hathorn Jacobson develop a book based on her diary entries, letters, and dictated material. Jacobson published the resulting work, *A Man Changes His Sex*, in Dutch and German in 1932 under the pseudonym Niels Hoyer. It was translated into English a year later as *Man into Woman: An Authentic Record of a Change of Sex* and is the first known book-length account of a gender transition.[128] Elbe was one of Hirschfeld's last patients. With the rise of Nazism, Hirschfeld's ability to do his work became increasingly difficult and then impossible after Adolf Hitler personally called Hirschfeld "the most dangerous Jew in Germany." Fearing for his life, Hirschfeld left the country. In his absence, the Nazis destroyed the institute in 1933, holding a public bonfire of its contents. Hirschfeld died in exile in France two years later.

In the US, Howard W. Jones pioneered intersex gynecologic surgery, by operating on babies with ambiguous genitalia (without the typical appearance of either a boy or girl), a practice that is now recognized as unacceptable. In 1965, he helped found the Johns Hopkins Gender Identity Clinic, the first sex-change clinic in an American hospital and performed the first gender change surgery on African American Phyllis Avon Wilson. The news of this made the gossip columns in 1966, the New York Daily News carried the item: "Making the rounds of the Manhattan clubs these nights is a stunning girl who admits she was male less than a year ago and that she underwent a sex change operation at, of all places, Johns Hopkins Hospital in Baltimore."

Later that year, The New York Times ran the story of the Gender Identity Clinic on the front page and announced the establishment of the Johns Hopkins Gender Identity Clinic under the chairmanship of plastic surgeon John Hoopes through a press conference. To an audience of 100 reporters, the doctors defined "transsexuals" (note, transexual as a term is not used anymore, transgender is) as "physically normal people who are psychologically the opposite sex," and explained that "psychotherapy has

---

[128] Hoyer, Niels, *Man Into Woman*, Popular Library, New York, 1953.

not so far solved the problem," and that they had already operated on 10 patients, all of whom were happy with the outcome.

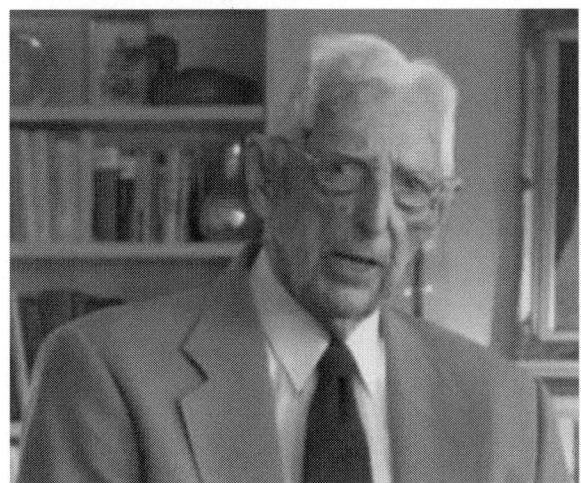

Image Source: Wikimedia Commons.
https://en.wikipedia.org/wiki/Howard_W._Jones.

Figure 14. Howard W. Jones, established the reproductive medicine center that was responsible for the birth of the first IVF baby in the U.S.

Sex Reassignmnet Surgery (SRS) are surgical procedures usually necessary for both Male to Female and Female to Male transgender individuals (trans) to reduce their distress caused by physical appearance. SRS is performed in 29-93% of trans people using different methods.[129] This intervention, which involves psychological, social, and legal aspects, is the most crucial step in changing the sexual characteristics of a trans individual to resemble those of another gender.[130] SRS in Male to Female trans involves implantation of breast prostheses, construction of a neovagina and clitoris, and other feminization surgeries. On the other hand, surgeries for Female to Male trans include hysterectomy with bilateral

---

[129] Toivonen KI, Dobson KS. Ethical issues in psychosocial assessment for sex reassignment surgery in Canada. *Can Psychol*. 2017;58(2):178.
[130] Sangganjanavanich VF. Sex reassignment surgery. In: Naples NA, editor. *The Wiley Blackwell encyclopedia of gender and sexuality studies*. 2016.

oophorectomy, development of the neophallus, and mastectomy.[131] SRS has been performed as part of the treatment of trans people for more than 70 years.[132] SRS has even been allowed as a treatment in Iran, since 1964.[133]

Sex reassignment surgery is the final step in the transition process. Comprehensive preoperative psychological and endocrinological evaluation and treatment are necessary before surgery. Initially, a person who is diagnosed with transgender identity (F64—according to the International classification of diseases— ICD -10) has to undergo a detailed assessment by two psychiatrists specialized in this field. This evaluation lasts for 6-12 months at least to obtain written consent to proceed with treatment (WHO, 2007). World Professional Association for Transgender Health (WPATH) published Standards of Care, which are designed for physicians, psychotherapists, social workers, and other specialists who work with trans people. Their goal is to achieve a permanent harmony with one's born identity safely and effectively, in order to improve their overall health, psychosexual and psychosocial aspects of life.[134]

Change from Female to Male Sex

Several surgical procedures can be done in female to male transgender, including mastectomy, removal of female genitalia, metoidioplasty, scrotoplasty with implantation of testicular implants, as well as total phalloplasty.

---

[131] Gooren LJ. Clinical practice. Care of transsexual persons. *N Engl J Med*. 2011;364(13):1251 7.
[132] Kuhn A, Bodmer C, Stadlmayr W, Kuhn P, Mueller MD, Birkhauser M. Quality of life 15 years after sex reassignment surgery for transsexualism. *Fertil Steril*. 2009;92(5):1685– 1689 e3.
[133] Hejazi A, Edalati Shateri Z, Mostsfsvi SS, Hoseyni ZS, Razaghiyan M, Moghadam M. [Assessment of compliance with gender roles and sexual identity 12 transsexual patients with new genders after sex reassignment surgery]. *J Kurdistan Univ Med Sci*. 2009;13:78– 87. Persian.
[134] Coleman E, Bockting W, et al. Standards of Care for the Health of Transsexual, Transgender, and Gender-Nonconforming People, Version 7. Int J Transgend, 2011;13:165– 232.

Change from Male to Female Sex

Several feminizing surgical procedures are performed in male to female transgender, including facial, neck, breast, and genital surgery. Genital reconstruction comprises vaginoplasty, introitoplasty, clitoroplasty, labiaplasty, and urethroplasty.

Gender identity influences every subjective aspect of life. Individuals with gender dysphoria face variable degrees of discrimination and traumatization because their gender expressions are not in line with the normative values of society. Individuals with gender dysphoria who have difficulty dealing with transphobia and public prejudice face numerous traumatic experiences in daily life. As a result, they may choose to hide their true feelings of gender. After gender reassignment surgery, many individuals prefer to live in a different social environment and protect their past.[135] Individuals with gender dysphoria have a greater possibility of being a victim of physical and verbal violence, have higher rates of unemployment, and are more prone to the risk of separation from their heterosexual partner.

They also have more feelings of loneliness in close relationships after the initiation of their gender reassignment procedure. Although the effects of adverse life events are different for everyone, research has shown that they are closely related to environmental circumstances. One study reported that fear of discrimination was related to symptoms of depression and anxiety.[136] Also, the attitudes of one's social networks and family are essential for mental health. It was found that transgender youth who felt that their self-respect was damaged by public prejudice and discrimination had increased rates of suicide.[137]

---

[135] De-Cuypere G, T'Sjoen G, Beerten R et al. (2005) Sexual and physical health after sex reassignment surgery. Arch Sex Behav 34:679–90.

[136] Fischer AR, Holz KB (2007) Perceived discrimination and women's psychological distress: The roles of collective and personal self-esteem. J Couns Psychol 54:154-64.

[137] Cole MC, O'Boyle M, Emory LE, Meyer WJ (1997) "Comorbidity of gender dysphoria and other major psychiatric diagnoses." Arch Sex Behav 26:13-6.

Although there is some recognition of the mental trauma associated with gender dysphoria, the majority of the articles about the effects of SRS on quality of life are usually about the medical consequences of the procedure.

BARRIERS TO SEX REASSIGNMENT SURGERY

Although there is overwhelming evidence that gender dysphoria is common and that surgical gender affirmation is an effective treatment for appropriately selected patients, there are strong cultural, religious, and even isolated academic opinions to the contrary. Among transgender people, rates of suicidal ideation and suicide attempts are high, homelessness as well as other hardships, like unemployment and poverty are faced. Many states have legislation that requires genital (sterilizing) surgery before transgender people can change their birth certificate, driver's license, and other identification documents. And voter identification laws can potentially disenfranchise an estimated 34,000 transgender people in local, state, and national elections.[138] Of note, transgender Americans are twice as likely as members of the general US population to serve in the US military. There are currently 134,300 transgender veterans and an estimated 15,000 transgender Americans in active military service.[139]

---

[138] Herman JL. "Strict voter ID laws may disenfranchise more than 34,000 transgender voters in the 2016 November election." Williams Institute. https://williamsinstitute.law.ucla.edu/research/strict-voter-id-laws-may-disenfranchise-more-than-34000-transgender-voters-in-the-2016-november-election/.

[139] Kauth MR, Blosnich JR, Marra J, Keig Z, Shipherd JC. Transgender health care in the US military and Veterans Health Administration facilities. *Curr Sex Health Rep*. 2017;9(3):121-127.

DENIAL OF GENDER-AFFIRMING CARE TO ARMED SERVICES VETERANS

Transgender patients and intersex individuals are provided with all care included in VA's (Veteran Affairs) medical benefits package, including but not limited to hormonal therapy, mental health care, preoperative evaluation, and medically necessary post-operative and long-term care following sex reassignment surgery to the extent that the appropriate health care professional determines that the care is needed to promote, preserve or restore the health of the individual and is in accord with generally-accepted standards of medical practice.

However, there has been the exclusion of gender-affirming surgery from the Health Benefits package that has been in place since 1992 in the US (National Center for Transgender Equality, 2017).

Due to a lack of understanding of SRS, it can be a stigmatizing and traumatic diagnosis for many. Often, physicians fail to understand the psychological ramifications of SRS for both the patient and the patient's family. Additionally, society struggles to accept those with SRS, as they do not fit into the ingrained sex binary. The sex binary is expressed in everything from public restrooms to bureaucratic forms. SRS conditions raise complex issues, including medicalization, parental acceptance, self-identity, and the production and dissemination of knowledge. SRS, which most times is advised as a result of the condition previously known as intersex conditions or hermaphroditism, is defined as a reproductive, genital, or chromosomal condition that deviates from the traditional definitions of male and female and occurs in up to 1:300 live births.

While the management of post-SRS has become more patient-centered than ever before, there remains significant stigmatization of SRS patients, perpetuated not only by society but also by the biomedical establishment. The most controversial aspect of SRS care is infant genital reassignment surgery, in which physicians surgically alter the external and/or internal genitalia to conform to society's definitions of female and male genitalia.

This surgery is medically unnecessary in the vast majority of cases because it is done for cosmetic reasons or to allow for penetrative intercourse.

Chapter 8

ASSISTED REPRODUCTIVE TECHNOLOGY

ASSISTED REPRODUCTIVE TECHNOLOGIES (ART)

Unlike Australia and England who have the Reproductive Technology Accreditation Committee (RTAC) and the Human Fertilization and Embryology Authority (HFEA) respectively to oversee assisted reproductive technology (ART), the USA lacks a centralized government healthcare system and financial oversight. In that vacuum, for better or worse, private *in vitro* fertilization (IVF) clinics have flourished. Highly publicized stories of accidents, and incidents of illegal, immoral, irresponsible, and unethical behavior, while they occur in every country, have fueled a notion in the US that ART is somehow a "wild west" medical specialty. Depending on who you ask, assisted reproduction is either *one of the most or least* regulated industries in the US.

Further fueling this speculation is the fact that the US is one of the only locations in the world where oocyte and sperm donation is not only legal but also relatively easy to accomplish. Additionally, gestational surrogates can be compensated well beyond just medical expenses. It is also legal for lesbian, gay, bi, trans, and queer (LGBTQ) people to pursue these options in the US. Unfortunately, that is not the case in many other countries, even in countries where gay marriage itself has been legal for a long time.

In the USA, IVF is a boutique industry, driven by consumer demand. In most parts of the country infertility is treated like a facelift or nose-job in luxurious clinics with crystal chandeliers, instead of as a critical medical procedure. Consumer demand also tends to drive the implementation of new techniques in ART in patients before large, well-designed clinical trials can confirm their safety and efficacy, such as cryopreservation of eggs, intracytoplasmic sperm injection (ICSI), embryo hatching, sex selection, cytoplasmic transfer, and preimplantation genetic diagnosis, among others.

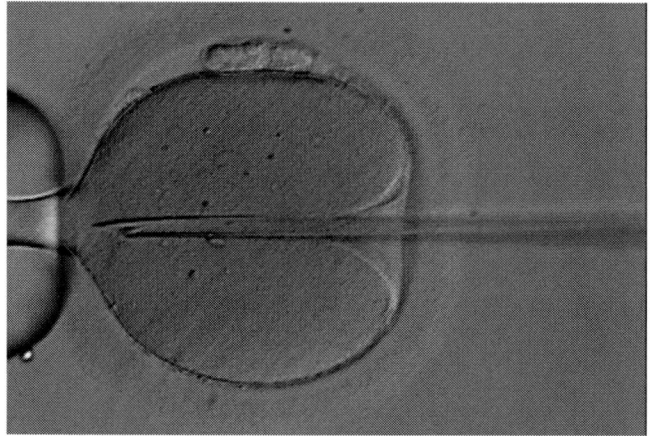

Image Source: Wikimedia Commons.
https://commons.wikimedia.org/wiki/File:ICSI.jpg.

Figure 15. A human oocyte is held by a glass holding pipette (left). A beveled glass pipette containing an immobilized ejaculated spermatozoon is inserted through the zona pellucida and deep into the oolemma.

Arkansas, California, Connecticut, Hawaii, Illinois, Louisiana, Maryland, Massachusetts, Montana, New Jersey, New York, Ohio, Rhode Island, Texas, and West Virginia have passed laws that require insurers to either cover or offer coverage for infertility diagnosis and treatment. More and more frequently, employers are recognizing that coverage of infertility services is very important to potential employees, as women in the workforce wait longer to start their families. Comprehensive, evidence-based infertility benefits can help attract and retain these top-talent and add very little to the bottom line.[140]

The regulation of ART in the US is fragmented, like many biotechnologies (genetic modification of organisms), and regulated by multiple agencies (Food and Drug Administration (FDA), Center for Disease Control (CDC) with overlapping or competing jurisdictions.

The regulation of IVF is complex because it involves the legal and ethical morass of creating human life, disposing of human embryos, compensating tissue donors (sperm and oocyte) and surrogates, and serving LGBTQ reproductive justice. But in fact, no other sub-specialty of medicine is required by federal law[141] to report its success rates to the US government. Over 95% of ART programs in the country annually report their results to the CDC through the Society for Assisted Reproductive Technology (SART), which has a contract with the CDC to collect these data. The federal government regulates all drugs and medical devices, as well as the reproductive tissue used in ART. The Clinical Laboratory Improvement Amendments of 1988 (CLIA 88) mandate certain standards for andrology laboratories and also cover those that provide ART services.

Professional societies and individual board certifications further enhance oversight of ART. The American Society for Reproductive Medicine (ASRM) was founded in 1944 and has been actively involved in research, education, and setting standards for practice in reproductive medicine, including ART. Founded in 1987, SART is an affiliate society of the ASRM; it published 1989 clinic-specific success rates on a voluntary basis and has continued annual publication since then. With the College of American Pathologists (CAP), SART, and ASRM also developed the CAP/ASRM Reproductive Laboratory Accreditation Programs (RLAP) that include strict standards for on-site laboratory inspections by CAP/ASRM/RLAP trained inspectors. At the state level, a license to practice medicine is required to practice ART, and most ART MD

---

[140] "Employers and Evidence-Based Fertility Benefits." https://resolve.org/wp-content/uploads/2017/09/employers-and-evidence-based-infertility-benefits.pdf.

[141] The United States is the Fertility Clinic Success Rate and Certification Act of 1992 (FCSRCA).

practitioners are certified by the American Board of Obstetrics and Gynecology, and many by the Reproductive Endocrinology Subspecialty Board. Facilities in which ART is practiced, such as hospitals, operating rooms, and procedure rooms, are subject to numerous regulations and licensing obligations.[142]

States are split about whether surrogacy contracts, usually between prospective parents and an oocyte donor, are permissible. Other aspects of ART are simply unaddressed. For example, states don't regulate how many children may be conceived from one donor, what types of medical information or updates must be supplied by donors, which genetic tests may be performed on human embryos, how many fertilized oocytes may be placed in a woman or how old a donor can be.

REPRODUCTIVE TISSUE DONATION

The US Centers for Disease Control and Prevention (CDC) publishes an annual report detailing the numbers, types, and success rates of infertility procedures in the US. From these data we know that the number of IVF cycles using donated eggs has jumped dramatically from just 1,802 cycles in 1992 to over 20,000 cycles in 2015.[143]

Like a dating website, oocyte donor websites display photos, medical histories, eye color, height, ethnicity or race, education level, personal interests, and family histories.

We know a lot about oocyte donor choice in infertile women, because some scientists have thought to ask the right questions. For example, we know that in the last decade, infertile women have started pursuing

---

[142] Adamson, David. "Regulation of assisted reproductive technologies in the United States," *Fertility and Sterility*, Vol. 78, Issue 5, p932-942, November 2002. https://www.fertstert.org/article/S0015-0282(02)04199-7/fulltext.

[143] "2015 Assisted Reproductive Technology National Summary Report," Centers for Disease Control. https://www.cdc.gov/art/pdf/2015-report/ART-2015-National-Summary-Report.pdf.

characteristics such as intelligence and athletic abilities over the appearance or genetic background of the oocyte donor.[144]

Due to availability (and legality) of tissue donation and surrogacy, LGBTQ individuals can now choose reproductive partners separately from the partners they engage in relationships with, and we have the opportunity to understand what the LGBTQ set of preferences for reproductive purposes are. These phenomena have been extensively studied in heterosexual individuals,[145,146] and the heteronormative set of standards for "physical attractiveness" informs the idealized images used in reproductive tissue advertising.[147]

Several studies have characterized the sexual attraction of some gay men to men in their late teens and early twenties, with physical attractiveness prioritized over status.[148,149] (Caution should be used, interpreting these results, as there are many sub-groups in gay culture, and these studies do not stratify based on sub group identification, and treat all gay men as if one belonging to one homogenous group.) There is very little published evidence examining gay intended parents' behaviors and choices with respect to either tissue donation or surrogacy. I could find just *one* abstract (from a conference proceeding[150]) that characterized the attitudes

---

[144] Flores, H, et all, "Beauty, Brains or Health: Trends in Ovum Recipient Preferences," Journal of Women's Health, Vol.23, NO. 10, October 2014. https://www.liebertpub.com/doi/full/10.1089/jwh.2014.4792.

[145] Townsend, J. M. (1989). Mate selection criteria: A pilot study. Ethology and Sociobiology, 10, 241–253.

[146] Townsend, J. M., & Levy, G. D. (1990). Effects of potential partners' physical attractiveness and socioeconomic status on sexuality and partner selection. Archives of Sexual Behavior, 19, 149–164.

[147] Richins, M. L. (1991). Social comparisons and the idealized images of advertising. Journal of Consumer Research, 18, 71–83.

[148] Kenrick, Douglas T., Keefe, Richard C., Bryan, Angela, Barr, Alicia, Brown, Stephanie. "Age preferences and mate choice among homosexuals and heterosexuals: A case for modular psychological mechanisms." *Journal of Personality and Social Psychology*, Vol 69(6), Dec 1995, 1166–1172

[149] Regan, P. C., Medina, R., & Joshi, A. (2001). "Partner preferences among homosexual men and women: What is desirable in a sex partner is not necessarily desirable in a romantic partner." *Social Behavior and Personality*, 29(7), 625–633.

[150] G. Sylvestre-Margolis, V. Vallejo, E. Rauch. Obstetrics and Gynecology, Flushing Hospital Medical Center, Flushing, NY; Obstetrics and Gynecology, RMA New Jersey, Freehold, NJ. "Gestational surrogacy / oocytedonor IVF: Behavior of gay men intended parents with

of very a small number of gay male intended parents with respect to the number of embryos transferred into their gestational carrier during a gestational surrogacy/oocyte donation IVF cycle.

While oocyte donation is a fairly new phenomenon in ART, sperm donation has a much longer history. The first sperm banks were instituted for the therapeutic purpose of infertility—one in Tokyo, Japan, and one in Iowa in 1964. The existence of sperm banks was made possible by enormous scientific advancements like the cryopreservation of human sperm with glycerol in 1949, and the first pregnancy conceived using thawed freezing sperm in 1953. In the US, more than a million people have been born with the help of sperm donation provided by commercial sperm banks in the last 40 years of operation.

Records of sperm donation goes back to at least 1785, when a Scottish anatomist and surgeon named Dr. John Hunter reported that he had successfully inseminated a woman based in London using her husband's sperm. A century later, the first Artificial Insemination (AI) on a woman was performed using donor sperm by Dr. William Pancoast in 1884. However, AI did not begin to become widely accepted until the 1940s when a need to repopulate after World War II and advances in birth control technology helped increase the popularity of the procedure. Most sperm banks initially began as non-profit, in-house clinics for male infertility treatment. Initially, these clinics used sperm only from their patients' husbands, storing and preserving the deposit for future use. Although the market for this service was little at the beginning, demand increased for donor sperm from women who either had an infertile husband, a husband with a genetic disorder, or no husband at all. Sperm banks gradually began to respond to this demand by accepting donations from men with no affiliation whatsoever with their patients, realizing in the process that there were several advantages to a more "objective system."

In the book *The Baby Business*, Professor Spar said by moving toward the market, seeking donors, and remunerating them a nominal fee, the clinics could shrink their reliance on their patients' sphere of friends, such

---

respect to number of embryos transferred." Abstract. *Fertility and Sterility*, October 20, 2015.

that a more anonymous type of quality control is created. The use of donated sperm gave women (and their husbands) the "opportunity" not to choose a *man* to father their child, giving them the liberty to only choose his sperm. Sperm donation is one of the oldest and most common procedures in assisted reproduction. Despite the lack of official data, in Greece more than forty private sperm banks offer cryopreserved sperm for *in vitro* fertilization (IVF) procedures. However, by the late 1980s commercial sperm banks had become a regular feature of the fertility sector, with over 400 clinics in operation. By 2009, commercial sperm banks were part of a $75 million per year industry, an excellent progression from the non-profit clinics that preceded them.

Sperm donation is allowed in 23 countries, however the laws governing it vary widely country to country.[151] Donor sperm are not allowed by law to be used for IVF in Austria, Germany, Italy, Tunisia, or Turkey. Donor perm must be obtained from specific registered banks in France, Norway, and Sweden. Only known donors may be used in the Netherlands, Norway, Sweden, and the United Kingdom, but only anonymous in Singapore, Slovenia, and Vietnam. Altruistic donors are required in Korea. In Switzerland, the recipients must be married, but single women and lesbians may be treated in the United Kingdom. In Taiwan, there must be no previous history of donation to achieve a live birth, and there are many other idiosyncrasies and variations across countries.

Today, the numbers of children that have been conceived by use of ART and donated gametes are increasing dramatically. Despite the reality that the use of donated sperm is one of the most ancient types of fertility treatment, it has traditionally been masked in secrecy, perhaps because it is most usually used to redress issues of a husband's infertility via the use of donated semen. In 1954, a US court ruled that donor insemination constituted adultery on the part of the woman, whether or not the husband

---

[151] Fertility and Sterility, Volume 87, Issue 4, April 2007. https://www.fertstert.org/article/S0015-0282(07)00258-0/pdf#:~:text=The%20use%20of%20donor%20sperm%20for%20other%20than%20IVF%20is,expenses%20are%20allowed%20in%20Greece.

had granted consent. Historically, unmarried women were prohibited from using AI because of conflicting societal norms; there was also a fear that unmarried women would not be able to adequately care for the child as a single parent.[152]

The debate over who can access IVF and what should be covered and for how long rages on to this day. In the US, we look to the UK's National Health Service (NHS) as a bastion of fair and equitable health coverage, yet the postcode lottery unfairly attacks single parents and assumes they will live in poverty and be a burden on the state and goes so far as to bar single women from obtaining IVF treatment coverage.[153] To this point, NHS published reprehensible comments that "Single mothers are generally poorer; they are likely to have greater support needs compared to two-parent couples."

ARTIFICIAL INSEMINATION

Artificial Insemination (AI) involves introducing sperm into a woman's uterus, vagina, or fallopian tubes with a needle to initiate a pregnancy. The sperm used in AI can be sourced from the woman's husband or a donor. The sperm can be fresh and used immediately or cryopreserved and stored for future use. A woman undergoing this procedure usually takes hormone medication that stimulates the ovaries to increase oocyte production in order to improve success rates. For males, especially, sperm donation is hardly an acceptable solution, as there is a complete separation between biological and social affiliation.[154] On the other hand, females consider sperm donation a less dramatic split; the

---

[152] Kritchevsky, Barbara. The Unmarried Woman's Right to Artificial Insemination: A Call for an Expanded Definition of Family, 4 Harv. Women's L.j. 1, 17 (1981)

[153] Pogrund, Gabriel. "NHS trusts deny single women IVF treatment." The Times. August 2019. https://www.thetimes.co.uk/article/nhs-trusts-deny-single-women-ivf-treatment-gs9b7qxbt

[154] David, G. (2000). Filiation in assisted reproduction with donor gametes. J. Gynecol. Obstet. (Paris), 29, 323±325.

genetic dissociation is partial, and the pregnancy creates and maintains a strong biological bond between child and mother.[155]

A systematic review of the literature concerning sperm donors isolated four different forms of motivation for donors: procreation, altruism, financial reward, and validation of personal fertility status.[156] Likewise, online donors have been reported to donate due to altruistic reasons though procreation was also considered as important.[157,158] The online donation also enables donors to donate while maintaining anonymity, such that recipients do not disclose the donor's identity to the resultant child, and in some cases, to the recipient.[159]

In 2009, William Marotta, from Topeka, Kansas, an auto-mechanic, answered a Craigslist Ad posted by Jennifer Schreiner and Angela Bauer, a lesbian couple in search of a private sperm donor for AI. After conferring the issue with his wife, Marotta organized an appointment with the lesbian couple and approved to donate. The parties then agreed to sign a contractual agreement intended to relieve Marotta of any future child support obligations and sever his parental rights. After the contract was signed, Marotta provided a sperm sample and delivered it in a plastic container to the couple's home. After this, he left. The couple then agreed that Schreiner would be the child's birthmother, and after just one attempt, the artificial insemination turned out successful and resulted in the birth of a baby girl. At no time during the process was a physician consulted. While Marotta's motivations were, in reality, altruist, what seemed to be a selfless act of benevolence brewed a risky legal situation. Kansas state

---

[155] David, G. (2000). Filiation in assisted reproduction with donor gametes. J. Gynecol. Obstet. (Paris), 29, 323±325.

[156] Van den Broeck U., Vandermeeren M., Vanderschueren D., Enzlin P., Demyttenaere K. and D'Hooghe T. A. (2013). :Systematic review of sperm donors: demographic characteristics, attitudes, motives and experiences of the process of sperm donation." *Hum Reprod Update* 2013;19:37–51.

[157] Freeman T., Jadva V., Tranfield E., and Golombok S. "Online sperm donation: a survey of the demographic characteristics, motivations, preferences, and experiences of sperm donors on a connection website." *Hum Reprod,* 2016;31:2082–2089.

[158] Woestenburg N. O. M., Winter H. B. and Janssens P. M. B. (2016). "What motivates Men to offer sperm donation via the internet?" *Psychol Health Med* 2016;21:424–430.

[159] Freeman T., Jadva V., Tranfield E., and Golombok S. "Online sperm donation: a survey of the demographic characteristics, motivations, preferences, and experiences of sperm donors on a connection website." *Hum Reprod,* 2016;31:2082–2089.

argued that because the insemination was not performed by a licensed doctor, the sperm donor contract was null and void, and the State fought him in court for more than four years about child support payment to the girl's mother after the couple filed for divorce.

In 2005, the UK eliminated donor anonymity signifying that all sperm donors who donate through a sperm bank or clinic registered with the Human Fertilization and Embryology Authority (HFEA) agree to their identifying information being made available to individuals born from their donation after they attain 18 years of age.[160] At the time the legislation came into force, there was concern about the possible effect this may have on donor numbers.

Intra-Family Sperm Donation

This involves the donation of sperm from a father or relation to another male within the family. There is evidence that the advanced male age may affect many sperm parameters. It has been reported that increased age is correlated with decreased semen volume, deteriorations in sperm morphology, and sperm motility.[161] Therefore, special attention has to be given to the health and the semen quality of the donors. But this may not be the trickiest part. The most severe risks are the emotional and ethical ones within the family circle.

Through Current Controversy

The capability of donor-conceived children to retrieve information concerning their genetic sources initially depends on their cognizance of the nature of their conception. Devoid of these facts, such children will

---

[160] Human Fertilisation and Embryology Authority (HFEA), (2004). *Disclosure of Donor Information. Regulations*. London: HFEA, 2004.
[161] Kidd, Sh.A., Eskenazi, B., and Wyrobek A.J. (2001). Effects of male age on semen quality and fertility: a review of the literature. Fertil. Steril., 75, 237±248.

presume that their "social" fathers are their genetic parents. Hence, the responsibility of disclosing the manner of conception lies on the social parents, except when such information is unveiled by the state, such as through a birth certificate, or it is evident that they cannot be the biological children of their social father. The advent of affordable DNA sequencing marketed directly to consumers[162] and social networks seeking to connect and support donor recipient families[163] effectively spell the end of guaranteed donor anonymity.

In the US some donor-conceived children are still grappling with the reality that the social father they have always known is not their genetic parent.[164] A now defunct practice called "confused insemination" allowed couples to mix donor sperm with the intended father's sperm, in order to keep alive the possibility that the child was biologically his. Couples were told by their doctor, to have intercourse before and after the procedure to further the sense that the (oftentimes completely sterile) husband could be the father. The subterfuge was even furthered as once a woman had become pregnant, the couple might be told that her blood levels showed she must have already been pregnant before the insemination, furthering the possibility that two otherwise rational people could believe their own narrative about the conception of their child.

As social views on same-sex relationships progress and reproductive technologies rapidly advance, the need for a clear perception of state parentage laws is imperative for all parties involved in assisted reproduction. One of the recurring issues that has engulfed courts in disagreements over parentage is whether the donor of sperm used for assisted reproduction is counted as a father, with full financial obligations and parental rights, or is considered as a donor, where financial obligations and parental rights can be severed. Several situations can emerge that give

---

[162] Keshavan, Meghana. "Consumer DNA Tests Negate Sperm-Bank-Donor Anonymity." STAT, September 2019. https://www.scientificamerican.com/article/consumer-dna-tests-negate-sperm-bank-donor-anonymity/
[163] https://donorsiblingregistry.com/
[164] Ridley, Jane. "I'm the result of a secret sperm concoction." *New York Post*, January 2019. https://nypost.com/2019/01/12/im-the-result-of-a-secret-sperm-concoction/

rise to legal concerns hinging on a genetic father's status as one or the other.

Legal Implications

The Uniform Parentage Act (UPA) of 1973 establishes paternity for children of married and unmarried couples. The Act created a way for the courts to identify a child's legal parents, regardless of marital status, and has been amended several times. The legal status of a sperm donor may turn on whether he is anonymous or non-anonymous, the sperm was given to a licensed physician or to the woman directly, the pregnancy was achieved using assisted reproductive technology, he and the woman had a pre-conception agreement with respect to parental status, and, in some situations, the development of a parent-child relationship after birth.

It was recently updated in 2017 to address the current use of reproductive tissue donation, ART, and legal same-sex marriage. It agrees that an individual may become a child's legal parent in any of the following ways:

- by giving birth to a child (aside from a gestational surrogate or a parent whose rights the court terminated),
- legally adopting a child,
- becoming a parent through another court process, or
- acknowledging paternity of the child.

Each state uses the UPA as a framework for developing ideal laws according to the state's policies and beliefs. States are free to accept all, none, or some of the provisions of the UPA. This has resulted in three-quarters of states with statutes based on the original 1973 UPA, some have been amended to reflect the emended changes, and some are completely unique. The natural consequence of this is that a majority of state courts still require physician involvement in artificial insemination in order for a paternal father to relinquish his paternity rights and to relieve him of child support obligations. In these states, cases in support of donor status when artificial insemination is performed at home are liable to fail, as courts are unenthusiastic to interpret the plain language of the 1973 UPA as anything but an absolute prerequisite that a physician is aboard.

Natural Insemination, or NI, is a term used to describe the process of a sperm donor inseminating a woman through sexual intercourse. It is often a method of surrogacy used when the intended parents don't have the funds to go through IVF and AI, as well as gives them more control in who they get to choose as a surrogate. The rise of the "natural insemination" industry is inevitably raising public health concerns—it is now being facilitated across the internet between private parties, is highly unregulated and certainly, it can be used disingenuously to simply meet other people to have unprotected sex with, and its potential for posing significant public health risks (through disease transmission or otherwise).

Another current ethical controversy is Posthumous Sperm Retrieval (PSR), a procedure of extracting spermatozoa from a human male after he has been pronounced legally brain dead. PSR gives rise to posthumous reproduction, either by artificial insemination or *in vitro* fertilization. In 1980, the first fruitful retrieval of sperm from a cadaver was reported, whereby a man became brain dead following an auto accident and whose family requested sperm preservation. Eight years later, the first successful conception by use of sperm retrieved post-mortem was achieved and reported, resulting in successful childbirth the following year. Over the years, there has been quite a number of important debates on the legality and ethicality of the procedure. The medical literature, however, recommends that extraction should be done within 24 hours after death; even as late as 36 hours after death, motile sperm have been successfully isolated regardless of the method of extraction or cause of death.

Most recently, the parents of an 18-year-old man who tragically died had his sperm posthumously retrieved, with the intent to carry out his wishes to have a family, despite him not having a romantic partner, and now being deceased.¹⁶⁵ The American Society for Reproductive Medicine (ASRM) had previously issued ethical guidelines in 2018 regarding posthumous collection of reproductive tissue. The guidelines say that it is justifiable if authorized in writing by the deceased. Otherwise, requests should only be considered from the surviving spouse or partner. In this case, the deceased had neither written documentation nor a partner. California Supreme Court Justice John Colangelo decided in the parents' favor, noting that, "At this time, the court will place no restrictions on the use to which Peter's parents may ultimately put their son's sperm, including its potential use for procreative purposes."

There is also the concern that half-siblings located near each other in a concentrated geographic area could increase the risk of accidental incest between half-brothers and half-sisters (inadvertent consanguineous conception). The issue is compounded by the fact that, although mothers of donor children are encouraged to report births, there is no requirement to do so. The US does not legally limit the number of offspring a sperm donor may produce, nor does it regulate anonymity. Numerous countries do restrict a donor's number of offspring, ranging from one (Taiwan) to 25 (the Netherlands). But the US and Canada have avoided legislating this, allowing for the possibility that half-siblings may inadvertently marry and have children. Again, ASRM offers guidelines suggesting a limit of six donations for oocyte donors, however they demur in limiting the number of sperm donations and simply say "that in a population of 800,000, limiting a single donor to no more than 25 births would avoid any significant increased risk of inadvertent consanguineous conception."¹⁶⁶

Laws should be enacted to relinquish the parental rights and obligations of the sperm donor such that people are encouraged to donate so those in need can have a child without fears of legal tussles for all parties. Along with the statutory enforcement of the written agreement between the donor and the recipient, there should also include an intent

---

¹⁶⁵ Drury, Cory. "Parents win right to use dead son's sperm so they can have grandchild." Independent. May 2019. https://www.independent.co.uk/news/world/americas/peter-zhu-death-frozen-sperm-parents-grandchild-surrogate-mother-a8924641.html.

¹⁶⁶ "Recommendations for gamete and embryo donation: a committee opinion." October 2012. https://www.fertstert.org/article/S0015-0282(12)02256-X/fulltext.

caveat which provides that the intent of the donor may override the enforceability of the written agreement. Societal and technological changes have allowed for a variety of options for creating familial relationships, such as gestational surrogacy and gamete donation. As technological and societal norms advance, the law often fails to progress. Non-traditional forms of creating a family call for new legal definitions of familial relationships.

ILLEGAL EMBRYOS

In 1952, two American embryologists, Robert Briggs and Thomas J. King,[167] became the first individuals to successfully clone an animal, by transferring the nuclei from early embryonic leopard frog cells into leopard frog oocytes that the nuclei had been removed from. Embryologists in other laboratories successfully repeated these initial experiments using different species of frogs. While the cells utilized were specialized, these cells were not obtained from the adult frog; in other words, these cells, in its real sense, may not have been fully differentiated.

The term "embryo" refers to the mass of cells in the most fundamental stages of its development into a new organism. The human embryo has been defined by scientists as the time starting from fertilization to the 8th week of gestation, which is 56 days from conception, the period when it becomes known as a fetus. This is the period when the embryo develops more advanced neurosensory and physical features begin.[168] Federal law in the US, however, does not define the term "embryo" explicitly; instead, it describes a fetus as the entity from the implantation stage (which scientists describe as 7–14 days from conception) to delivery.

Due to continuous early human embryo research, IVF became a success, a development that revolutionized medical treatment for

---

[167] Briggs, R., and King, T. J. (1952). "Transplantation of living nuclei from blastula cells into enucleated frog's eggs," Proceedings of the National Academy of Sciences (USA) 38: 455-463, 1952.
[168] Sadler, Thomas W. (2015). Langman's Medical Embryology. Philadelphia: Wolters Kluwer.

infertility. Scientists worked for decades, improving IVF techniques before it was first carried out successfully in 1978 by two British Scientists, Robert Edwards, and Patrick Steptoe.[169] This manipulation of human embryos in the lab and successful birth of the world's first IVF baby, Loise Brown, was greeted as both a revolution for infertile couples and horror at the great "leap into the unknown." It was predicted that "all hell would break loose, politically and morally all over the world" and assembly line fetuses would be grown in test tubes like plants in a nursery.

Of course, those fears never came to pass, and to date millions of IVF babies have been born worldwide. Human embryo research received significant attention from the media again when it was connected to the budding field of regenerative medicine. In 1998, scientists, many of whom were from the United States, reported culturing human embryonic stem cells (hESCs) for the first time.[170] These cells are obtained from five- to six-day-old embryos and presented scientists the possibility of producing virtually any tissue or cell in the human body. The promise of hESCs as novel tools to study the most basic human development and several disease states to ultimately acquire treatments to replace injured or diseased tissues and/or cells is tempered with the means of acquisition of them. The isolation of these embryonic cells requires the destruction of human embryos.

Even before IVF was first successfully carried out in 1978, discussions were underway in the US over whether research that uses embryos or results in their destruction is ever permissible and, if so, under what circumstances.[171] Since the first-ever successful IVF procedure in 1978, the application of this and associated technologies has become normalized all

---

[169] Johnson, Martin H. "Robert Edwards: the path to IVF." Reproductive biomedicine online vol. 23,2 (2011): 245-62. doi:10.1016/j.rbmo.2011.04.010 https://www.ncbi.nlm.nih.gov/pmc/articles/PMC3171154/.

[170] Thomson, James A., Joseph Itskovitz-Eldor, and Sander S. Shapiro (1998). "Embryonic Stem Cell Lines Derived from Human Blastocysts." Science 282, no. 5391: 1145–47. http://science.sciencemag.org/content/282/5391/1145.long.

[171] Kass, Leon R. (1971). "Babies by Means of *in vitro* Fertilization: Unethical Experiments on the Unborn?" New England Journal of Medicine 285, no. 21: 1174-79.

over the world.[172] Over the past decade, Assisted Reproduction Technology (ART) services usage has surged at a pace of 5 - 10% yearly.[173,174] The birth of Dolly the Sheep in 1997 was an extraordinary scientific accomplishment, which fundamentally altered the way biologists view the control of genetic information in animal cells. It revealed a greater than expected capacity to "reprogram" cells, to reset the genetic program that guides development. But Dolly's birth correspondingly unleashed worries about human cloning, and these fears have limited the quest for a promising way of cell reprogramming for therapeutic uses.

What is human cloning? This is simply the asexual production of a new human organism, which at all levels of development is genetically practically identical to an either previously existing human being or currently living person. Human cloning can be achieved by introducing the nuclei of a human somatic cell (which is the donor) into an oocyte (ovum) whose own nucleus has been either inactivated or removed. Thus, giving up a product that has a human genetic composition practically identical to the somatic cell donor. (This technique is known as "somatic cell nuclear transfer.")

3-Person Embryos

In 1997, the first live birth from an embryo that contained the DNA of three different people, which had been created through "ooplasm transfer" was reported.[175] It was thought at the time that this scientific feat would be celebrated and the technique would be considered similar to any other

---

[172] Steptoe, P. C., and Edwards, R. G. (1978). "Birth after the reimplantation of a human embryo," The Lancet, vol. 2, no. 8085, p. 366, 1978.
[173] Chambers, G. M., Sullivan, E. A., Ishihara, O., Chapman, M. G., and Adamson, G. D. (2009). "The economic impact of assisted reproductive technology: a review of selected developed countries." Fertility and Sterility, vol. 91, no. 6, pp. 2281–2294, 2009.
[174] Thomson, James A., Joseph Itskovitz-Eldor, and Sander S. Shapiro (1998). "Embryonic Stem Cell Lines Derived from Human Blastocysts." Science 282, no. 5391: 1145–47. http://science.sciencemag.org/content/282/5391/1145.long.
[175] "Recommendations for gamete and embryo donation: a committee opinion." October 2012. https://www.fertstert.org/article/S0015-0282(12)02256-X/fulltext.

treatment involving donated organs, oocytes, or cells. No one suspected that this would cause a regulatory nightmare, but it did. Regulatory agencies were furious, claiming that the researchers were genetically engineering human embryos and immediately halted the practice. That is because mitochondria (organelles inside cells that are inherited in oocyte cytoplasm) have their own separate DNA, which carries 13 genes total. Another live birth from a "3-person" embryo would not occur until 2016, when the New Hope Fertility Center in New York announced the birth of a baby boy, followed by a baby girl in the Ukraine in 2017.

An embryo that contains DNA from three different people can be created in one of three ways: pronuclear transfer, maternal spindle transfer, or nuclear genome transfer. Pronuclear transfer uses a one-day-old embryo created from the parents' sperm and oocyte and replaces its nucleus into another pronuclear stage embryo that has been made with a donor's oocyte and the father's sperm. The result is an embryo made up of nuclear chromosomes from the parents containing 99.9 percent of the DNA, and healthy mitochondrial DNA from a donor woman. Maternal spindle transfer involves replacing the nucleus of a donor oocyte with a nucleus removed from one of the mother's oocytes. Nuclear genome transfer is performed with unfertilized oocytes.

The technique can be used for couples that want a biological child of their own, but who would pass on a sometimes-fatal mitochondrial genetic disorder. Unhealthy mitochondria can cause severe medical disorders that affect the heart, kidney, skeletal muscle, and brain. More controversially, this technique is thought to be able to reverse some of the oocyte ageing that makes it more difficult for older oocytes to make successful embryos that can result in live, healthy births. Fertility clinics in the US have been reprimanded for marketing this unproven technique to patients.[176]

---

[176] https://www.fda.gov/media/106739/download.

Genetic Engineering Human Embryos

Two Chinese infants, Lulu and Nana, hold the distinction of being the world's first CRISPR gene edited children. CRISPR stands for clustered regularly interspersed short palindromic repeats. Correcting genetic defects in humans (genetic engineering or gene surgery) is a rapidly developing technology that can save tens of millions of lives and provide dramatically better quality of life to hundreds of millions. In 2018, Chinese scientist He Jiankui flouted the international scientific community by announcing the birth of the twin girls and gestation of a third gene edited embryo. The flaws and ethical lapses in his work were many: inadequate medical indication, a poorly designed study protocol, a failure to meet ethical standards for protecting the welfare of research subjects, and a lack of transparency in the development, review, and conduct of the clinical procedures.

"Gene surgery" may not be viewed as another IVF procedure now, but undoubtedly it will be in the future. He used the CRISPR Cas system to edit the genes of embryos that would become Lulu and Nana. The CRISPR/Cas9 was adapted to genome editing in 2013.[177] Since then, molecular biologists have edited genes with unprecedented accuracy and speed. The prokaryotic-clustered, regularly interspaced, short palindromic repeats (CRISPR) loci were first characterized in 1993, and it was subsequently discovered that they were part of the bacterial "adaptive" immune system. Animal and plant genomes can be edited (genetically modified) using a single enzyme called Cas9, to introduce CRISPR derived RNAs at double-stranded DNA breaks.[178] Recent studies have shown that Cas9 and engineered single guide RNAs (sgRNA) are the only components

---

[177] Cong L, Ran FA, Cox D, Lin S, Barretto R, Habib N, Hsu PD, Wu X, Jiang W, Marraffini LA, Zhang F. "Multiplex genome engineering using CRISPR/Cas systems." Science. 2013;339(6121):819–23. doi: 10.1126/science.1231143. PubMed PMID: 23287718; PMCID: PMC3795411.

[178] Wiedenheft B, Sternberg SH, Doudna JA. "RNA-guided genetic silencing systems in bacteria and archaea." Nature. 2012;482(7385):331–8. doi: 10.1038/nature10886. PubMed PMID: 22337052.

necessary and sufficient for efficient genome editing in cultured human cells, mouse and rat, fruit flies, worms, and fish.

The first transgenic animals were produced more than 30 years ago, and today the majority of transgenic animals are produced by microinjection of plasmid DNA into the pronuclei of fertilized oocytes. CRISPR/Cas9 replaces older, slower, costlier and labor-intensive genetic engineering methods: plasmid, bacterial artificial chromosomes, yeast artificial chromosomes, zinc fingers, and transcription activator-like effector nuclease (TALENs).

In other words, CRISPR/Cas9 lends itself to high efficiency and scaled production of transgenic and genome edited organisms. Almost any gene can be easily added or modified in any organism imaginable.

In the US, the National Institutes of Health (NIH) refuses to even fund research into gene-editing technologies in human embryos, despite its tremendous potential. The arguments against human genetic engineering are based on social stigmas arising from the fear of the unknown, driven largely by religious ideology and anti-science rhetoric.

"The truth is humanity has always engaged in genetic modifications," said former president Barack Obama.[179]

Nearly all bans on research prove to be temporary, as science eventually tends to trump politics. There is a high cost to human lives when we allow fear, religious ideology, and superstition to delay the development and application of life saving technologies. Recently, in acknowledgment of the CRISPR/Cas9 developments and need to apply this technology to human well-being, the National Academy of Science, Engineering, and Medicine developed seven general principles for the governance of human genome editing.

---

[179] starting around 2:13:22, https://www.youtube.com/watch?v=1yBJHQ-jMUY&feature=emb_logo.

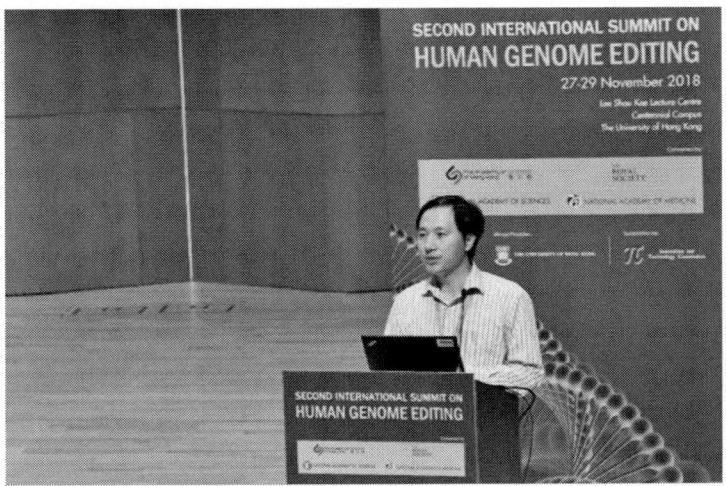

Image Source: Wikimedia Commons.
https://commons.wikimedia.org/wiki/File:He_Jiankui_at_Summit_on_Human_Genome_Editing,_Hong_Kong.png.

Figure 16. He Jiankui, a Chinese biophysics researcher, announces birth of genetically engineered human babies at the Summit on Human Genome Editing on 28 November 2018 in Hong Kong.

There are several arguments against genetic engineering of human embryos:

- *We are our genes. Altering that changes who we "should be" fundamentally:* Is there anything inherently wrong with genetic modification? Is the human genome sacred? This is an argument from genetic reductionism/fatalism, i.e., that a person is determined by his/her genes. This argument is used by some people who feel that even if we do modify human genes, it should only be for the sake of disease prevention or treatment and not for "enhancement." No reputable geneticist or psychologist believes that we are solely determined by our genes. Our gene's potential is only realized in our environment. For example, even if a parent wanted to confer some amazing genetic trait—let's say fast twitch muscle fiber so they could win Olympic-level track and field events—it would still be up to that child to practice that skill, eat right, train every day, mentally train for, and make the Olympics. A genetic advantage (being "naturally good" at something) may even be a detriment, if the person decides to rest on their genetic laurels and put in less effort than they should.

- *Genetically engineered children would be commodities:* As with any new reproductive technology, such as, sperm donation, *in vitro* fertilization, and surrogacy, opponents claim that they might create children who are potentially "unlovable." This argument is absurd of course, as it is often *conventional* reproduction that creates hundreds of thousands of accidental and unloved children.
- *Genetic engineering of humans could reduce biological diversity:* Genetic engineering is simply a tool. It could be used with the motive of creating uniformity, but it would certainly fail, unless you genetically modified every single person on earth, for the exact same trait, at the exact same instant, and then "de novo" mutations could not occur. This scenario is simply put, impossible. Not only that, but who is to say that it would not be used for the opposite reason, to try to increase diversity? This would also fail since populations tend to "regress to the mean." In our thought experiment; pink, blue, green, and purple skinned humans would all breed together and regress to the mean color.
- *Genetically engineered humans would be considered "less-human":* It is a principle of ethics that the origins of a person do not affect their "personhood." That's how we got eugenics as a shameful legacy. The correct response to prejudice is to expose it for what it is, combat it with reason and evidence, not validate it as an ethical reason to not do something.
- *People created by genetic engineering may be used for spare parts or organs:* Nothing could be done to a person created with genetic engineering that right now could not be done to your brother or to a person's twin. The US Constitution strongly implies that once a human fetus is outside the womb and alive, it has autonomous bodily rights. No matter what its method of production or state of

being. We can't even use organs from a dead person without their consent.
- *Human genetic engineering is inherently evil:* To most people the words "genetic engineering" or "genetic modification" are packed with bad connotations—implying selfish motives, crazy scientists, and out-of-control technology. It is none of those things, but simply a tool. We should call it something neutral or even something with a positive connotation such as "gene-editing."

Human genetic engineering could be risky: We don't know every possible pitfall of CRISPR/Cas9 technology, nor can we. Pregnancy and reproduction in general are extremely risky, oftentimes resulting in stillbirth, genetic defects, congenital defects, and more. If "no risk" was a condition of making babies then deaf people would not be allowed to have babies together, for example. Women would not be allowed to have unmonitored home births. Fertility drugs would not be allowed. Women over 40 or under 16 wouldn't be allowed to get pregnant, but none of these things are true. People take calculated and even unnecessary risks in pregnancy and childbirth all the time.

- *Only selfish people would genetically engineer or create a "designer" baby:* Is it selfish to "design" a baby? This is a question that no one, including our government has the right to ask. Several Supreme Court decisions declare that all forms of human reproduction, including the right not to reproduce, cannot be abridged by the government. Our government must not ever require, or judge, any couple's reasons for having a child, even if they are seen by others to be selfish.
- *Scientists who work on human genetic engineering are evil or motivated by bad motives:* From Icarus to Frankenstein to Boys From Brazil to Jurassic Park and today's Stranger Things, scientists and engineers throughout time have been portrayed as hubristic, evil, or working for corrupt governments. Coercive eugenics and associated ideas of state-mandated population genetic engineering as a form of social control morally unacceptable for

any genetic or reproductive technology and are not specific to genetic engineering. Scientists are just people. Most of them have kids of their own and care a lot for kids.

- *Embryos can't give consent:* "Embryos cannot decide for themselves whether to undergo genome editing; they are unable to give consent and have no choice over the alterations inflicted upon them." This holds true for any child conceived by any method. Likewise, you cannot force a woman to have a chromosomal screening, or to not carry a genetically defective fetus to term.

The ability to easily create genetically modified organisms raises profound questions about ourselves, our practice of science, and even our ability to alter the character of our world and all of humanity. Just as there has been a rush to condemn human cloning, and before that human *in vitro* fertilization, there has been a rush to condemn genetic modification in general, despite its proven safety record, and especially, genetic modification of humans.

Ethical Concerns Related to Human Cloning

- Problems of identity and individuality: The expectations for their lives might be stalked by the constant appraisal of the life of the "prototype."
- Concerns regarding manufacture: Concerns about "creating children for commercial and industrial purposes.
- The prospect of a new eugenics. The possibility, someday in the future, of using cloning to perpetuate genetically engineered enhancements.
- Troubled family relations: By transgressing and confounding the natural boundaries among generations, human cloning could inevitably strain the social ties. Genetic relation to just one parent could create other inconveniences for family life.

- Effects on society: Even if performed on a small level, it could alter the manner society views children.

PERSONHOOD BILLS

In 2008, Kristi Burton, a homeschooled college student, almost single-handedly got a ground-breaking measure that defines a constitutionally protected person as "any human being from the moment of fertilization," onto the Colorado state ballot. Ultimately, voters rejected the measure, but since then, wave after wave of so called "Personhood" bills have been put forth on state ballots.

Embryo research is critical to human health and well-being and the advancement of medical therapies; for example, to solve the problem of miscarriage which affects 1 out of every 4 pregnancies, to understand the causes and cures for developmental disorders (congenital anomalies), or how viral infections impact pregnancy and fetal development, to name just a few.

On August 23, 2010, a federal district court judge issued an injunction blocking federal funding for research on embryonic stem cells. The judge ruled that federal funding would violate a 1996 law (the so-called Dickey Amendment) which prohibits funding of research that results in the destruction of embryos or subjects' embryos to a risk of injury.

People who oppose embryo research hold the belief that an embryo (a grouping of cells less than 14 days old) should have the same rights as an adult human being.

There are many flaws in this reasoning. Consider that between two-thirds and four-fifths of all embryos that are generated through standard sexual reproduction are spontaneously aborted–and we now know through the advent of preimplantation genetic testing that a significant number of human embryos are genetically flawed. If embryos have the same status as human persons, this would be a horrific aberration—but no one treats this as a vast public health crisis. No one would suggest marshaling all of our public health resources and funding to "solve" this problem.

The early embryo is not an individual. Until about 14 days after conception, the embryo can divide into two or more parts. Under the right conditions, each of those parts can develop into a separate fetus.

The potential of the embryo does not make it a human person. Those who rely on the potential of the embryo to support their claim that it is morally equivalent to an adult human conveniently ignore the important role that women and wombs play in embryonic and fetal development. An embryo in a petri dish is not capable of becoming a fetus. It requires nutrients provided by the mother through the placenta in order to develop into a fetus, and we don't even understand all necessary factors to maintain pregnancy.

Additionally, relevant to this discussion, is the fact that embryos used for research are spare embryos from *in vitro* fertilization (IVF) procedures. In other words, they are embryos that are destined for the waste basket, unless they are used in research. They have no prospect of developing into a fetus.

Chapter 9

RESEARCH AND DEVELOPMENT

HUMAN REPRODUCTIVE EXPERIMENTATION

The history of IVF is steeped in controversial human experimentation and research. In their quest to be the first to create a successful human pregnancy from a laboratory grown embryo, IVF pioneers Robert Edwards and Patrick Steptoe conducted experiments on 282 women who underwent a total of 495 failed IVF cycles. Could they have known the risks and limitations of the procedures?[180] Sandra Crashley, a patient of Steptoe's, describes in her book, *My Ordeal in Edward's Nobel Prize: The Testimony of an IVF Guinea Pig,* the removal of one-and-a-half of her ovaries without her permission. A procedure she says shocked her body into early menopause and rapid aging. To this day, although millions of babies have been born through IVF, the cost remains steep, and the success rates remain lower than we would like. Current controversies surround everything from pricey "add-ons" with unclear effectiveness,[181] to oocyte freezing,[182] to extremely controversial "ovarian rejuvenation therapy" with

---

[180] Zoll, Miriam. "Questioning the Cult of Repro Tech." The Dark Mountain Project. October 2015. https://dark-mountain.net/questioning-the-cult-of-repro-tech/.
[181] "IVF add-ons: the latest Cochrane evidence. October 2020. https://www.evidentlycochrane.net/ivf-add-ons-the-latest-cochrane-evidence/.
[182] Bearne, Suzanne. "Single women are paying thousands to freeze their eggs – but at what cost?" The Guardian. March 2019. https://www.theguardian.com

PRP (plasma rich in platelets) ovarian "injury"—therapies that are undergoing clinical trials,[183] but are directly marketed to the consumer[184] despite evidence of effectiveness.

The control of reproduction or cure for infertility has always been highly sought after. Surgeon John Romulus Brinkley is best known for implanting men with goat testicles in an attempt to cure impotence. Brinkley was able to reach large audiences with the help of the newly popular radio station. He operated on many men over the years, taking in thousands of dollars. His unprofessional and unethical escapades prompted the authorities to seize his medical license and radio license, in an effort to end his sham surgeries in 1930.

Dr. Landrum Shettles reportedly carried out the first known clinical IVF procedure in the USA. Shettles covertly arranged a course of IVF treatment for private patients Doris and John Del-Zio in 1973, which was interrupted prior to embryo transfer by Shettle's senior colleague Raymond Vande Wiele. A month later, Shettles was forced to resign, and the Del-Zios sued the hospital, and eventually won a modest settlement for "intentional infliction of emotional distress." Shettles later became known for his shoddy and ill supported by scientific evidence theories of sex selection (that x and y bearing sperm swam differently), and later opening a failed "human cloning" clinic in Las Vegas.

Like many other scientists and physicians of the day, the legacy of Howard W. Jones is unequivocally is of a pioneer who changed the lives of millions through his work, but is complicated by what we now view as violating patient informed consent and performing experimental human surgeries without knowing the risks and consequences. He is the surgeon responsible for the infant-intersex surgeries (then called 'corrective' surgery) that lead to great harm (such as the suicide of David Reimer), but in 1965 he also pioneered and performed the first surgery on their

---

/science/2019/mar/23/single-women-are-paying-thousands-to-freeze-their-eggs-but-at-what-cost.

[183] https://clinicaltrials.gov/ct2/show/NCT04444245

[184] Sipp, Douglas, et al. "Marketing of unproven stem cell-based interventions: A call to action." Science Translational Medicine 05 Jul 2017: Vol. 9, Issue 397, eaag0426 https://stm.sciencemag.org/content/9/397/eaag0426.short

transgender patients starting with Phyllis Avon Wilson at the Gender Identity Clinic at Johns Hopkins Hospital (Chapter 7). Howard also established the cytogenetics laboratory at Johns Hopkins when the field was in its infancy and was the first physician at Johns Hopkins to examine Henrietta Lacks (Chapter 1).

More recently, a group of reproduction researchers has conducted a somewhat controversial study that involved remunerating dozens of young ladies at a hospital close to Puerto Vallarta, Mexico, to hyper stimulate the ovaries, inseminate them artificially, then flush out the resulting embryos before they could implant in the uterus. As a result, their embryos can be flushed out of their bodies then analyzed for research purposes[185]. The method aims to make embryos that are of satisfactory or better quality compared to those created through IVF, says reproductive geneticist Santiago Munne, who headed the study. A feat that many others consider as unethical research. Ethicist Laurie Zoloth, from the University of Chicago, considers this research to be profoundly disturbing, essentially using a woman's body as a petri dish.

This avenue of research has been undertaken in order to offer couples with genetic abnormalities, who are at risk of transmitting them to their offspring, the ability to select embryos that are not affected. It can also offer couples a less expensive method of having healthy children, unlike generally expensive IVF. This technique could also be useful for lesbian couples such that birth partners can have each participate in a pregnancy, one by donating oocytes and the other carrying the pregnancy.

Although the study technically passed IRB approval, it doesn't sit well with many people. It raises some serious ethical concerns. For example, these women were paid close to $1,400, which is equivalent to more than two month's average wages paid to workers in the area where this study was conducted. Furthermore, a number of the women had to undergo chemical/surgical abortion afterward, as subsequent tests showed that some of the embryos were not removed successfully.

---

[185] Munné, Santiago et al. First PGT-A using human *in vivo* blastocysts recovered by uterine lavage: comparison with matched IVF embryo controls. Hum Reprod. 2020 Jan; 35(1): 70–80. https://www.ncbi.nlm.nih.gov/pmc/articles/PMC6993848/.

This research was the first-time human embryos were created naturally but analyzed with preimplantation genetic diagnostic tests to see if they are abnormal or normal. Despite the seemingly utopian probabilities this research wishes to address, it raises a series of concerns, including ethical, social, and legal perspectives.

CHIMERAS—HOW MUCH HUMAN DNA IS TOO MUCH?

Genetic and embryo engineering (blastocyst complementation techniques) have made the generation of part-human chimeras possible, but also raises difficult questions about the moral status of creatures that are neither fully animal nor fully human. Hybrid embryos are distinct from chimeric embryos; they are embryos that have been created by the fertilization of a human oocyte by animal sperm, the fertilization of an animal oocyte by human sperm, or via nuclear transfer between animal and human eggs. Chimera research is important, as it can be used to generating human organs in animals, we typically already butcher for the food supply, provide transplantable organs that can circumvent the need for (and burdens of) lifelong immunosuppression; to better study heritable human diseases, and find drugs that work against these diseases.

Scientists have added human brain genes to macaque monkeys[186] and made a mouse embryo that was composed of 4% human cells (highest amount yet).[187] In Japan scientists recently mixed human cells into mouse and rat embryos, then transplanted those embryos into surrogate mothers until they developed close to term but they terminated the pregnancies before live birth.[188]

---

[186] Burrell, Teal. "Scientists Put a Human Intelligence Gene Into a Monkey. Other Scientists are Concerned." Discover Magazine. December 2019. https://www.discovermagazine.com/mind/scientists-put-a-human-intelligence-gene-into-a-monkey-other-scientists-are.

[187] Hu, Zhixing, et al. "Transient Inhibitor of mTor in human pluripotent stem cells enables robust formation of mouse-human chimeric embryos." *ScienceAdvances Magazine.* May 2020. https://advances.sciencemag.org/content/6/20/eaaz0298.

[188] Cryanoski, David. "Japan approves first human-animal embryo experiments. Nature. July 2019. https://www.nature.com/articles/d41586-019-02275-3.

Table 2. International legislation part-human chimeric embryos

Australia	The Prohibition of Human Cloning for Reproduction Act prohibits the creation of chimeric embryos via the introduction of animal cells into human embryos, but not via the introduction of human cells into animal embryos.
Canada	The Assisted Human Reproduction Act 2004 prohibits the creation of chimeras, which are defined as (human) embryos into which cells from other animals or humans have been introduced; it does not prohibit the creation of chimeric embryos by introducing human cells to animal embryos. However, the main agencies responsible for funding scientific research in Canada expressly prohibit the creation of either form of chimeric embryo, effectively blocking any such research.
USA	Although federal laws do not restrict the creation of part-human chimeras, the National Institutes of Health has issued a moratorium on federal funding for human-animal chimera research as it considers ethical issues associated with the introduction of human stem cells to animal embryos.
UK	The Human Fertilisation and Embryology Act 2008 prohibits keeping a human admixed embryo for longer than 14 days or beyond the appearance of the primitive streak, as well as placing a 'human admixed embryo' in an animal to develop.
Germany	The Embryo Protection Act 1990 prohibits the creation of chimeras via introducing animal cells to a human embryo or fusing human and animal embryos.
International guidelines	The International Society for Stem Cell Research (ISSCR) Guidelines for Stem Cell Research and Clinical Translation recommend that part-human chimera research should not be pursued if it involves breeding part-human chimeras with the potential to form human gametes. The guidelines also hold that research involving chimerism of either the central nervous system or germ line should be subject to specialized research oversight to address possible animal welfare issues.

Research science is grappling with questions like: How much human DNA or cells is too much? How "far away" evolutionarily does a research animal have to be, to combine human genes or cells with it? How long can chimeras be grown, in the lab and after transplantation to surrogate mothers? Concluding in some cases, such as in "The ethics of using transgenic non-human primates to study what makes us human,"[189] that human brain genes should never be added to apes, such as chimpanzees, because they are too similar to us. Legislative approaches[190] seek to answer these questions mainly by considering the possibility of substantial moral status of any chimera containing human cells.

14 Days: The Limit of Human Life in the Lab

Two laws—one in the US[191] and one in the UK[192]—have shaped the viewpoint worldwide called the "14-day rule." The 14-day rule for embryo research stipulates that laboratory experiments with intact human embryos must not allow them to develop beyond 14 days or the appearance of the primitive streak. In the past, embryos rarely grew beyond day 5, 6, or, at the upper limit, 7 days in the lab, before stalling out and degenerating. On day 7, human embryos naturally implant in the wall of the uterus. So, the 14-day rule was mainly a theoretical and philosophical limit. The implantation time-period is essential for pregnancy. Early miscarriage is a devastating and intractable problem. Understanding the early placenta and other cell types that support embryonic growth is imperative to make advances.

However, recent advances in cell culture techniques, such as the discovery of certain growth factors necessary for human embryos to

---

[189] Coors, Marilyn E et al. "The ethics of using transgenic non-human primates to study what makes us human." Nature reviews. Genetics vol. 11,9 (2010): 658-62. doi:10.1038/nrg2864 https://pubmed.ncbi.nlm.nih.gov/20717156/.

[190] Julian J Koplin, Julian Savulescu, Time to rethink the law on part-human chimeras, Journal of Law and the Biosciences, Volume 6, Issue 1, October 2019, Pages 37–50, https://doi.org/10.1093/jlb/lsz005 https://academic.oup.com/jlb/article/6/1/37/5489767.

[191] HEW Support of Research Involving Human *in Vitro* Fertilization and Embryo Transfer: Report and Conclusions, Ethics Advisory Board (1979)

[192] Report of the Committee of Inquiry Into Human Fertilisation and Embryology, M Warnock (1984)

"implant" on the bottom of a culture dish without the need for maternal tissues[193] have now cast that 14-day limit into the limelight.

Additionally, another team from the University of Michigan, recently coaxed human stem cells to make structures that resemble early embryos. They developed a microfluidic system that produces embryo-like structures, known as synthetic human entities with embryo-like features (SHEEFs) with a primitive streak—one of the least understood events in early human development. The reason why we know so little about the development of the primitive streak is because it develops in embryos before many women know they are pregnant but just after the time limit that human embryos can legally grow in a laboratory. Should such groupings of cells fall within the 14-day rule?

So why 14-days? The Warnock Committee cited possible sentience (the ability to feel pain) and individuation (the emergence of a definite single human individual) as the main reasons. The commission noted that "neural development begins at around 17 days" and that "subtracting a few days" from this would ensure "that there would be no possibility of the embryo feeling pain."[192]

Ethical and evidence-based policy is now needed because the 14-day limit avoids precisely those processes that are important to normal embryonic development (epiblast expansion, lineage segregation, bi-laminar disc formation, amniotic and yolk sac cavitation, and trophoblast diversification).

PROCURING FETAL TISSUE FOR RESEARCH

Fetal tissue used for research is primarily obtained from elective abortions, which women can consent to donate after deciding to terminate a pregnancy. There are only two choices, throw this tissue away or use it for invaluable medical research.

---

[193] Shahbazi, Marta N et al. "Self-organization of the human embryo in the absence of maternal tissues." Nature cell biology vol. 18,6 (2016): 700-708. doi:10.1038/ncb3347 https://pubmed.ncbi.nlm.nih.gov/27144686/.

Table 3. Federal funding of research involving human embryos and fetuses[194]

Fetal research	Allowed in accordance with 1974 law and subsequent regulations, which prohibit researchers from having any involvement in the decision to terminate a pregnancy or assessing fetal viability and forbid altering the timing or method of abortion for the sake of research and the payment of any inducements that might encourage a woman to have an abortion.
Fetal tissue transplantation research	Allowed in accordance with 1993 law, which ensures informed consent, forbids the woman providing the tissue from being paid or knowing the identity of the recipient, forbids altering the timing or method of abortion for the sake of research and attempts to avoid the commercialization of fetal tissue.
In vitro fertilization research	Effectively prohibited by 1995 law, which blocks funding for any research in which human embryos are destroyed, discarded, or knowingly subjected to serious risk.
Stem cell research	Allowed in some cases in accordance with 1993 law. Strict National Institutes of Health guidelines permit the use only of cells derived from excess embryos that had been created for fertility treatments and otherwise would be discarded; research involving stem cells derived by cloning may not be funded. Funding for the actual derivation of stem cells from embryos is prohibited by 1995 law (see *In vitro* fertilization research, above).

Research involving fetal tissue has been a mainstay of modern medicine, funded in large part with federal dollars without controversy. Dating back to the 1930s, scientists have used tissue from aborted fetuses as a means of understanding cell biology and as an important tool in the development of vaccines. The 1954 Nobel Prize for Medicine, for example, was awarded to American immunologists who developed the polio vaccine based on cultures of human fetal kidney cells. However, in 1988, former US President Ronald Reagan placed restrictions on federal funding for fetal tissue studies, which stayed in place until President Bill Clinton overturned them during the first year of his term in 1993. President

---

[194] Boonstra, Heather D. "Human Embryo and Fetal Research: Medical Support and Political Controversy." Guttmacher Institute. February 2001. https://www.guttmacher.org/gpr/2001/02/human-embryo-and-fetal-research-medical-support-and-political-controversy.

Donald Trump's administration tried to reenact those restrictions, including banning government scientists from using this fetal tissue for research and applying increased scrutiny for National Institutes of Health (NIH) grant proposals from nongovernmental scientists.

The Open Philanthropy Project[195] is a nonprofit organization that seeks to use private donors to shore up research funding when the US political climate gets more restrictive. But nonprofits are not the only option. In California, the state's stem cell agency, the California Institute for Regenerative Medicine (CIRM), has provided funding for stem cell studies using fetal tissue since it was founded in 2004.

---

[195] https://www.openphilanthropy.org/.

REFERENCES

Auer TO, Del Bene F. CRISPR/Cas9 and TALEN-mediated knock-in approaches in zebrafish. *Methods.* 2014;69(2):142–50. doi: 10.1016/j.ymeth.2014.03.027. PubMed PMID: 24704174.

Barbara Kritchevsky (1981). *The Unmarried Woman's Right to Artificial Insemination: A Call for an Expanded Definition of Family*, 4 Harv. Women's L.j. 1, 17 (1981).

Bassett AR, Tibbit C, Ponting CP, Liu JL. Highly efficient targeted mutagenesis of Drosophila with the CRISPR/Cas9 system. *Cell Rep.* 2013;4(1):220–8. doi: 10.1016/j.celrep.2013.06.020. PubMed PMID: 23827738; PMCID: PMC3714591.

Briggs, R., and King, T. J. (1952). "Transplantation of living nuclei from blastula cells into enucleated frog's eggs," *Proceedings of the National Academy of Sciences* (USA) 38: 455-463, 1952.

Brown, K. (1995). "Changed ... into the fashion of man": The politics of sexual difference in a seventeenth-century Anglo-American settlement. *Journal of the History of Sexuality*, 6 (21), 171-93.

Chambers, G. M., Sullivan, E. A., Ishihara, O., Chapman, M. G., and Adamson, G. D. (2009). "The economic impact of assisted reproductive technology: a review of selected developed countries." *Fertility and Sterility*, vol. 91, no. 6, pp. 2281–2294, 2009.

Cho SW, Kim S, Kim JM, Kim JS. Targeted genome engineering in human cells with the Cas9 RNA-guided endonuclease. *Nat Biotechnol.* 2013;31(3):230–2. doi: 10.1038/nbt.2507. PubMed PMID: 23360966.

Cole MC, O'Boyle M, Emory LE, Meyer WJ (1997) Comorbidity of gender dysphoria and other major psychiatric diagnoses. *Arch Sex Behav* 26:13-6.

Coleman E, Bockting W, et al. Standards of Care for the Health of Transsexual, Transgender, and Gender-Nonconforming People, Version 7. *Int J Transgend,* 2011;13:165– 232.

Cong L, Ran FA, Cox D, Lin S, Barretto R, Habib N, Hsu PD, Wu X, Jiang W, Marraffini LA, Zhang F. Multiplex genome engineering using CRISPR/Cas systems. *Science.* 2013;339(6121):819–23. doi: 10.1126/science.1231143. PubMed PMID: 23287718; PMCID: PMC3795411.

Cromwell, J. (1999). *Transmen and FTMs: Identities, bodies, genders, and sexualities.* Urbana: University of Illinois Press.

David, G. (2000). Filiation in assisted reproduction with donor gametes. *J. Gynecol. Obstet.* (Paris), 29, 323±325.

De-Cuypere G, T'Sjoen G, Beerten R et al. (2005) Sexual and physical health after sex reassignment surgery. *Arch Sex Behav* 34:679–90.

Fertility Clinic Success Rate and Certification Act of 1992 (FCSRCA), Pub. L. no. 102 —493,1992.

Fischer AR, Holz KB (2007) Perceived discrimination and women's psychological distress: The roles of collective and personal self-esteem. *J Couns Psycholm* 54:154-64.

Freeman T., Jadva V., Tranfield E. and Golombok S. (2016) Online sperm donation: a survey of the demographic characteristics, motivations, preferences, and experiences of sperm donors on a connection website. *Hum Reprod,* 2016;31:2082–2089.

Friedland AE, Tzur YB, Esvelt KM, Colaiacovo MP, Church GM, Calarco JA. Heritable genome editing in C. elegans via a CRISPR-Cas9 system. *Nat Methods.* 2013;10(8):741–3. doi: 10.1038/nmeth.2532. PubMed PMID: 23817069; PMCID: PMC3822328.

Gooren LJ. Clinical practice. Care of transsexual persons. *N Engl J Med.* 2011;364(13):1251 7.

Gordon JW, Scangos GA, Plotkin DJ, Barbosa JA, Ruddle FH. Genetic transformation of mouse embryos by microinjection of purified DNA. *Proc Natl Acad Sci USA.* 1980;77(12):7380–4. PubMed PMID: 6261253; PMCID: PMC350507.

Gratz SJ, Cummings AM, Nguyen JN, Hamm DC, Donohue LK, Harrison MM, Wildonger J, O'Connor-Giles KM. Genome engineering of Drosophila with the CRISPR RNA-guided Cas9 nuclease. *Genetics.* 2013;194(4):1029–35. doi: 10.1534/genetics.113.152710. PubMed PMID: 23709638; PMCID: PMC3730909.

Hejazi A, Edalati Shateri Z, Mostsfsvi SS, Hoseyni ZS, Razaghiyan M, Moghadam M. [Assessment of compliance with gender roles and sexual identity 12 transsexual patients with new genders after sex reassignment surgery]. *J Kurdistan Univ Med Sci.* 2009;13:78–87. Persian.

Herman JL. *Strict voter ID laws may disenfranchise more than 34,000 transgender voters in the 2016 November election.* Williams Institute. https://williamsinstitute.law.ucla.edu/research/strict-voter-id-laws-may-disenfranchise-more-than-34000-transgender-voters-in-the-2016-november-election/.

Hsu PD, Scott DA, Weinstein JA, Ran FA, Konermann S, Agarwala V, Li Y, Fine EJ, Wu X, Shalem O, Cradick TJ, Marraffini LA, Bao G, Zhang F. DNA targeting specificity of RNA-guided Cas9 nucleases. *Nat Biotechnol.* 2013;31(9):827–32. doi: 10.1038/nbt.2647. PubMed PMID: 23873081; PMCID: PMC3969858. http://science.sciencemag.org/content/282/5391/1145.long.

Human Fertilisation and Embryology Authority (HFEA), (2004). *Disclosure of Donor Information. Regulations.* London: HFEA, 2004.

Jaenisch R, Mintz B. Simian virus 40 DNA sequences in DNA of healthy adult mice derived from preimplantation blastocysts injected with viral DNA. *Proc Natl Acad Sci USA.* 1974;71(4):1250–4. PubMed PMID: 4364530; PMCID: PMC388203.

Jain, T., and Hornstein, M. D. (2005). "Disparities in access to infertility services in a state with mandated insurance coverage," *Fertility and Sterility*, vol. 84, no. 1, pp. 221–223, 2005.

Jones, H. W., Cooke, I., Kempers, R., Brinsden, P., and Saunders, D. (2011). "International Federation of fertility societies surveillance," Fertility and Sterility, vol. 95, no. 2, p. 491, 2011.

Julie E. Goodwin (2005). *Not All Children Are Created Equal: A Proposal to Address Equal Protection Inheritance Rights of Posthumously Conceived Children*, 4 conn. *Pub. Int. L.j.* 208, 212, (2005).

Kansas *ex rel.* Sec'y Dep't for Children & Families v. W. M., Case No. 12 D 2686 (Kan. Dist. Ct. Jan. 22, 2014) (memorandum decision and order granting petitioner's motion for summary judgment).

Kass, Leon R. (1971). "Babies by Means of *in vitro* Fertilization: Unethical Experiments on the Unborn?" *New England Journal of Medicine* 285, no. 21: 1174-79.

Kauth MR, Blosnich JR, Marra J, Keig Z, Shipherd JC. Transgender health care in the US military and Veterans Health Administration facilities. *Curr Sex Health Rep*. 2017;9(3):121-127.

Kidd, Sh. A., Eskenazi, B., and Wyrobek A. J. (2001). Effects of male age on semen quality and fertility: a review of the literature. *Fertil. Steril.*, 75, 237±248.

Kirstin R. W. Matthews and Erin H. Yang (2019). *Drawing The Line Politics And Policies Guiding Human Embryo Research In The United States.* January 2019.

Kuhn A, Bodmer C, Stadlmayr W, Kuhn P, Mueller MD, Birkhauser M. Quality of life 15 years after sex reassignment surgery for transsexualism. *Fertil Steril*. 2009;92(5):1685–1689 e3.

Li D, Qiu Z, Shao Y, Chen Y, Guan Y, Liu M, Li Y, Gao N, Wang L, Lu X, Zhao Y, Liu M. Heritable gene targeting in the mouse and rat using a CRISPR-Cas system. *Nat Biotechnol*. 2013;31(8):681–3. doi: 10.1038/nbt.2661. PubMed PMID: 23929336.

Mojica FJ, Diez-Villasenor C, Garcia-Martinez J, Soria E. Intervening sequences of regularly spaced prokaryotic repeats derive from foreign genetic elements. *J Mol Evol.* 2005;60(2):174–82. doi: 10.1007/s00239-004-0046-3. PubMed PMID: 15791728.

Mojica FJ, Juez G, Rodriguez-Valera F. Transcription at different salinities of Haloferax mediterranei sequences adjacent to partially modified PstI sites. *Mol Microbiol.* 1993;9(3):613–21. PubMed PMID: 8412707.

National Center for Transgender Equality. *ID documents center.* https://transequality.org/documents, 2018.

National Center for Transgender *Equality. Issues: military and veterans.* http://www.transequality.org/issues/military-veterans, 2017.

Office of tech. Assessment, US Cong., *OTA-13p-ba-48, artificial insemination practice in the United States: summary of a 1987 survey—background paper 8-9 (1988)*, available at http://www.fas.org/ota/reports/8804.pdf.

Papadopulos NA, Lelle JD, Zavlin D, Herschbach P, Henrich G, Kovacs L, et al. Quality of life and patient satisfaction following male to female sex reassignment surgery. *J Sex Med.* 2017;14(5):721–30.

Pourcel C, Salvignol G, Vergnaud G. CRISPR elements in Yersinia pestis acquire new repeats by preferential uptake of bacteriophage DNA, and provide additional tools for evolutionary studies. *Microbiology.* 2005;151(Pt 3):653–63. doi: 10.1099/mic.0.27437-0. PubMed PMID: 15758212.

Sadler, Thomas W. (2015). *Langman's Medical Embryology*. Philadelphia: Wolters Kluwer.

Sander JD, Joung JK. CRISPR-Cas systems for editing, regulating and targeting genomes. *Nat Biotechnol.* 2014;32(4):347–55. doi: 10.1038/nbt.2842. PubMed PMID: 24584096; PMCID: PMC4022601.

Sangganjanavanich VF. Sex reassignment surgery. In: Naples NA, editor. *The Wiley Blackwell encyclopedia of gender and sexuality studies.* 2016.

Steptoe, P. C., and Edwards, R. G. (1978). "Birth after the reimplantation of a human embryo," *The Lancet*, vol. 2, no. 8085, p. 366, 1978.

The President's Council on Bioethics Washington, DC. *Human Cloning and Human Dignity: An Ethical Inquiry.* July 2002. www.bioethics.gov.

Thomson, James A., Joseph Itskovitz-Eldor, and Sander S. Shapiro (1998). "Embryonic Stem Cell Lines Derived from Human Blastocysts." *Science* 282, no. 5391: 1145–47.

Toivonen KI, Dobson KS. Ethical issues in psychosocial assessment for sex reassignment surgery in Canada. *Can Psychol.* 2017;58(2):178.

Tzur YB, Friedland AE, Nadarajan S, Church GM, Calarco JA, Colaiacovo MP. Heritable custom genomic modifications in Caenorhabditis elegans via a CRISPR-Cas9 system. *Genetics.* 2013;195(3):1181–5. doi: 10.1534/genetics.113.156075. PubMed PMID: 23979579; PMCID: PMC3813848.

US Department of Veterans Affairs Veterans Health Administration. *VHA Directive 2013-003 Providing health care for transgender and intersex veterans.*

Van den Broeck U., Vandermeeren M., Vanderschueren D., Enzlin P., Demyttenaere K. and D'Hooghe T. A. (2013). Systematic review of sperm donors: demographic characteristics, attitudes, motives and experiences of the process of sperm donation. *Hum Reprod Update* 2013;19:37–51.

Wendy Moore (2005). *The Knife Man: The extraordinary life and times of John Hunter, father of modern surgery* (2005).

WHO International Statistical Classification of Diseases and Related Health Problems, 10th revision, Geneva, Switzerland, 2007.

Wiedenheft B, Sternberg SH, Doudna JA. RNA-guided genetic silencing systems in bacteria and archaea. *Nature.* 2012;482(7385):331–8. doi: 10.1038/nature10886. PubMed PMID: 22337052.

Wierckx K, Van Caenegem E, Pennings G, Elaut E, Dedecker D, Van de Peer F, et al. Reproductive wish in transsexual men. *Hum Reprod.* 2012;27(2):483–7.

Woestenburg N. O. M., Winter H. B. and Janssens P. M. B. (2016). What motivates Men to offer sperm donation via the internet? *Psychol Health Med* 2016;21:424–430.

ABOUT THE AUTHOR

Carol Lynn Curchoe Burton is a renowned scientist, and those suffering from infertility in the fight against infertility, and to educate and excite the general public about science and cutting-edge technologies, such as; cloning, embryonic stem cell research, artificial intelligence, IVF, embryology and more. She enjoys being a special guest for podcasts, keynote lectures, presentations, and collaborations.

Her PhD in the physiology of reproduction is from the University of Connecticut and she is board certified as a technical supervisor of embryology. She is the founder of ART Compass, (www.artcompass.io) a mobile application platform for IVF cycle management, a Fertility Guidance Technology (www.fertilityguidancetechnologies.com).

INDEX

#

14-day rule, 124, 125

A

abortion, xv, xvi, 10, 25, 27, 28, 29, 30, 46, 57, 58, 59, 79, 80, 121, 126
abortion pill, 30
abortion reversal, 59
abstinence-only sex education, 24
American College of Obstetrics and Gynecology, 11
American College of Radiology, 40
Anderson, Lucy Hicks, 74
anesthesia, 3, 5, 7, 8, 9, 12, 47, 50
artificial insemination (AI), ix, 1, 98, 100, 101, 104, 105, 129, 133
assisted reproduction, xvi, 61, 93, 99, 100, 101, 103, 109, 130
assisted reproduction technology, 61, 109

B

Baartman, Saartjie (Sarah), 17
Barnum, P. T., 19
Belmont Report, 14
Briggs, Robert, 107
Brinkley, John Romulus, 120
Buck v. Bell, 23, 41

C

California Institute for Regenerative Medicine (CIRM), 127
Cartwright, Samuel, 5
chemical castration, 43, 44
childbirth, 6, 10, 47, 48, 49, 51, 52, 53, 58, 78, 83, 105, 115
chimeras, ix, 122, 123, 124
Comstock Acts, 21
confused insemination, 103
consent, xvi, 4, 8, 9, 10, 11, 12, 14, 20, 23, 25, 28, 42, 43, 50, 52, 53, 57, 60, 63, 76, 88, 100, 115, 116, 120, 125, 126
Contagious Diseases Act, viii, 33
conversion therapy, viii, 76, 77, 78
Couney, Martin, 20
crisis pregnancy centers, 57

CRISPR, 111, 112, 115, 129, 130, 131, 132, 133, 134
C-sections, 49, 50, 52
Cuvier, Baron known as Cuvier, Georges, 19

D

Dickey Amendment, 117
Dolly the Sheep, 109

E

Edwards, Robert, 108, 119
Elbe, Lili, 84
emergency contraception, 26, 27
endometriosis, xii, 7
episiotomy, viii, 48, 49, 51, 83
eugenics, vii, 21, 22, 35, 41, 114, 115, 116

F

female genital mutilation (FGM), xii, 81, 83
female reproductive tract, 65, 66, 68, 69, 73
fistula, vii, 1, 3, 49
Frédéric, Jean Léopold Nicolas, 19

G

gay marriage, 93
gender dysmorphia, 45
gender identity, 72, 76, 78, 86, 89, 121
gender parity, 12
gender-affirming surgery, xvi, 91
genital cutting, viii, 81, 82, 83
genital transformation surgeries, 84
Gey, George O., 12
Goedken, Jennifer, 9
gonadal dysgenesis, 72
Griswold v. Connecticut, 24

Griswold, Estelle, 24
Guevedoces, 70
gynecology, i, ii, iii, xii, 1, 2, 8, 12, 45, 48, 96, 97

H

Halley, Edmond, 16
HeLa, vii, xii, 12, 13, 14, 60
Henrietta Lacks, vii, 12, 13, 14, 15, 60, 121
Heth, Joice, 19
hormonal contraception, 11
Hottentot Venus, 18
human cloning, 109, 116, 120, 123, 133
human embryonic stem cells (hESCs), 108
human embryos, 95, 96, 108, 110, 111, 112, 113, 117, 122, 123, 124, 125, 126
human zoos, vii, 15, 17
husband stitch, viii, xvi, 53
Hyde Amendment, 27
hysterectomy, 11, 46, 63, 87
hysteroscopy, 7

I

ice bucket challenge, 20
in vitro fertilization (IVF), xiii, 59, 79, 87, 93, 94, 95, 96, 97, 98, 99, 100, 105, 107, 108, 111, 114, 116, 118, 119, 120, 121, 126, 135
indigenous peoples, 16, 17
infant incubator, 20
infant mortality, 59, 63
infertility, xi, xiii, 36, 38, 59, 61, 62, 63, 94, 95, 96, 98, 99, 108, 120, 132, 135
intersex, viii, 76, 81, 83, 86, 91, 120, 134
intrauterine devices (IUDs), 25

J

Johns Hopkins, 12, 13, 14, 86, 121
Johns Hopkins Gender Identity Clinic, 86
Jones, Howard W., 86, 87, 120

K

King Louis XIV, 48
King, Thomas J., 107

L

Landrum Shettles, 120
LGBTQ, 77, 93, 95, 97
live autopsies, 20

M

male circumcision, 81, 82
male reproductive tract, viii, 65, 66, 69, 73
maternal fetal death rate, 49
maternal spindle transfer, 110
Mayer-Rokitansky-Küster-Hauser, 70
menstrual hygiene products, 30, 31
midwifery, 55, 57
Müllerian ducts, 67, 68, 69
Müllerian Inhibiting Substance, 69
Museum of Man in Paris, 19

N

Native American, 17, 42
Natural History Museum in London, 16
natural insemination, 105
Newton, Isaac, 16
NIFLA v. Becerra, 57
Noeggerath, Emil, 33

O

Obama, Barack, 15, 112
obstetric trauma, 55
obstetrics, 1, 8, 12, 45, 48, 53, 57, 96, 97
oocyte donor, 96, 106
oral birth control pills, 21
ovaries, 13, 39, 66, 69, 72, 75, 85, 100, 119, 121

P

pain management, 6, 7
pelvic exam, vii, xvi, 8, 9, 10, 11, 12
pelvic inflammatory disease, 7
pelvic rehabilitation, 10
period poverty, vii, 30
personhood bills, ix, 117
Petiver, James, 16
pink tax, 31
Plan B, 26, 27
Planned Parenthood, xv, xvi, 21, 22, 23, 28
Planned Parenthood v. Casey, xv, xvi, 28
posthumous reproduction, 19, 105
posthumous sperm retrieval, 105
postnatal PTSD, 48
primordial gonads, 67
public dissection, 20

R

Rebecca Gomperts, 30
reproductive justice, 3, 30, 95
Reproductive Laboratory Accreditation Programs (RLAP), 95
Reynolds v. Reynolds, 37
Roe v. Wade, xv, xvi, 28
Röntgen, Wilhelm Conrad, 39

S

Sanger, Margaret, xvi, 21, 22, 23
sex binary, 91
sex selection, viii, 78, 79, 80, 94, 120
sexual health, 10, 12, 25, 35, 60, 62
shackling of pregnant prisoners, 53
Sims, J. Marion, 1, 2, 4, 22
slavery, 5, 16, 17
Society for Assisted Reproductive Technology (SART), 95
somatic cell nuclear transfer, 109
speculum, vii, 1, 3, 5
sperm banks, 98, 99
sperm donation, 93, 98, 99, 100, 101, 102, 106, 114, 130, 134
spermist theory of reproduction, 66
SRY (sex related gene), 68, 69, 71
steatopygia, 18
Steptoe, Patrick, 108, 119
stereotypes (racial and gender), 7
sterility, 2, 33, 96, 98, 99, 109, 129, 132
sterilization laws, 41, 60
surgical castration, viii, 43, 44
surrogacy, 36, 96, 97, 105, 107, 114
symphysiotomy, 49, 50

T

testicles, 39, 66, 70, 73, 120
The American Society for Reproductive Medicine (ASRM), 95, 106
The Family Planning Services and Public Research Act of 1970, 42
the pill, 23, 24, 25, 30

third sex, 75
Title X Family Planning Program, 42
tourist transplant, 15
transatlantic slave trade, 16
transgender, 74, 75, 78, 86, 87, 88, 89, 90, 91, 121, 130, 131, 132, 133, 134
TRAP laws, 29
tubal ligations, viii, 45, 46
Turing, Alan, 44
turnaway study, 59

U

Uniform Anatomical Gift Act, 19

V

vasectomy, 45
vice reform, 34

W

Whole Woman's Health v. Hellerstedt, 28
Wolffian ducts, 67, 68

X

X chromosome, 70, 73
X-rays, 39, 40

Y

Y chromosome, 68, 70, 71